Interpreting
Electrocardiograms

FUNDAMENTAL AND CLINICAL CARDIOLOGY

Editor-in-Chief
Samuel Z. Goldhaber, M.D.
*Harvard Medical School
and Brigham and Women's Hospital
Boston, Massachusetts*

Associate Editor, Europe
Henri Bounameaux, M.D.
*University Hospital of Geneva
Geneva, Switzerland*

ADDITIONAL VOLUMES IN PREPARATION

Interpreting
Electrocardiograms
Using Basic Principles and Vector Concepts

J. Willis Hurst

Emory University School of Medicine
Atlanta, Georgia

MARCEL DEKKER, INC.   NEW YORK · BASEL

ISBN: 0-8247-0513-0

This book is printed on acid-free paper.

Headquarters
Marcel Dekker, Inc.
270 Madison Avenue, New York, NY 10016
tel: 212-696-9000; fax: 212-685-4540

Eastern Hemisphere Distribution
Marcel Dekker AG
Hutgasse 4, Postfach 812, CH-4001 Basel, Switzerland
tel: 41-61-261-8482; fax: 41-61-261-8896

World Wide Web
http://www.dekker.com

The publisher offers discounts on this book when ordered in bulk quantities. For more information, write to Special Sales/Professional Marketing at the headquarters address above.

Series Introduction

Marcel Dekker, Inc., has focused on the development of various series of beautifully produced books in different branches of medicine. These series have facilitated the integration of rapidly advancing information for both the clinical specialist and the researcher.

My goal as editor-in-chief of the Fundamental and Clinical Cardiology series is to assemble the talents of world-renowned authorities to discuss virtually every area of cardiovascular medicine. In the current monograph, *Interpreting Electrocardiograms: Using Basic Principles and Vector Concepts*, J. Willis Hurst has written a much-needed and timely book. Future contributions to this series will include books on molecular biology, interventional cardiology, and clinical management of such problems as coronary artery disease and ventricular arrhythmias.

Samuel Z. Goldhaber

Preface

This book should be viewed as an introduction to the subject of electrocardiography. The book is for clinicians who intend to use the electrocardiogram as a *diagnostic tool*, not merely a recording completed to conform to recommended practice guidelines. The basic principles used to interpret cardiac arrhythmias are different from those used to interpret abnormalties of the P waves, QRS complexes, S-T segments, and T waves, and for this reason they are not discussed here. This book deals only with the basic principles used to determine the direction and size of the electrical forces that produce the P, QRS, S-T, and T waves.

Much has been learned recently about the mind and how it works (1). We now better understand where we register images in our brains, how we store the images to create a memory, and how we use the stored memories to think and learn. This new knowledge about the mind, plus the knowledge gained from fifty years of teaching, have led me to conclude that few individuals can memorize huge numbers of electrocardiographic patterns and become fluent in the interpretation of them. Accordingly, *the basic principles of electrocardiography that are needed to understand the shapes of the waves are presented here, along with the admonition that they must be used to interpret every electrocardiogram.* If memorization must be done, I suggest that the basic principles be memorized—don't hurdle over them to memorize the shapes of waves in an effort to find a shortcut to learning.

The basic principles discussed in this book should be stored in the brain; I refer to them as images or memories. They should be used in the thinking process that is required to interpret each electrocardiogram. Normal and abnormal electrocardiograms are then viewed within the context of basic principles.

The brilliant electrocardiographer Frank Wilson said it this way in 1952 (2):

> The interpretation of the electrocardiogram is not merely a matter of memorizing a few characteristic pictures; there are many unusual variations and combinations of electrocardiographic phenomena which must be studied, analyzed, and correlated one with another and with other available data before any definite conclusion is possible. *These situations demand some acquaintance with the electrical and physiologic principles by which they are determined.*

Lord Kelvin emphasized that an individual who intends to collect scientific information about any subject must measure. He wrote the following in the late 1800s (3):

> When you can measure what you are speaking about, and express it in numbers, you know something about it; but when you cannot measure it, when you cannot express it

in numbers, your knowledge is of a meager and unsatisfactory kind: it may be the beginning of knowledge, but you have scarcely, in your thoughts, advanced to the stage of *science*.

This leads us to the use of vector concepts as a method of thinking about and understanding the waves in the electrocardiogram. Whereas vectors were used by Waller, Einthoven, and Wilson to represent the electrical forces of the heart, and many others in explaining the waves, Grant and Estes popularized the method of using vector concepts to interpret each electrocardiogram (4). Accordingly, the method of Grant is discussed and used in this book.

I wish to acknowledge the help of Carol Miller in the preparation of this manuscript. She is a genius at deciphering my "pen scratching" on a sheet of paper and translating it into legible type.

I thank my wife, Nelie, for tolerating the disarray created in our home by my writing binges. The preparation of this sally of words was especially messy because to write this book I pulled together several decades of accumulated papers and illustrations. So, I say once again: no Nelie—no book.

J. Willis Hurst

REFERENCES

1. Carter R. *Mapping the Mind*. Berkeley: University of California Press, 1998.

2. Wilson F. N. Foreword. In: Barker J. M. *The Unipolar Electrocardiogram: A Clinical Interpretation*. Appleton-Century-Crofts: New York, 1952, pp. xi–xii.

3. William Thomson, Lord Kelvin. *Popular Lectures and Addresses 1891–1894*.

4. Grant R. P., Estes E. Jr., *Spatial Vector Electrocardiography*. Philadelphia: The Blakiston Company, 1951.

Acknowledgments

Most of the illustrations used in this book were published earlier in the following books: Hurst & Woodson, *Atlas of Spatial Vector Electrocardiography*, The Blakiston Company, 1952; Hurst & Wenger, *Electrocardiographic Interpretation*, McGraw-Hill, 1963; Hurst & Myerburg, *Introduction to Electrocardiography*, McGraw-Hill, 1973; Silverman, Myerburg, & Hurst, *Electrocardiography: Basic Concepts and Clinical Application*, McGraw-Hill, 1983. The publishers returned the copyright of these books to me. For simplicity, I have cited the original source of the illustrations even though many of them appeared in several of the books listed above. I have also used illustrations from the following more recently published books.

Hurst: *Ventricular Electrocardiography*, Gower Medical
   Publishing, 1991. The publisher returned the copyright to me. This book also appears on the Internet
   (Medscape), but I retained the rights to the material.
Hurst: *Cardiovascular Diagnosis: The Initial Examination*, Mosby, 1993. The publisher returned the copyright to me.

   I thank my friends and patients, Mack and Grace Worden
of Clearwater, Florida, for their support in the production of
this book.

Contents

About the Author

J. WILLIS HURST is a Consultant to the Division of Cardiology, Emory University School of Medicine, Atlanta, Georgia, where he was professor and chairman of the Department of Medicine from 1957 to 1986. The author or coauthor of more than 60 books, including *Clinical Neurocardiology* (Marcel Dekker, Inc.), and nearly 400 articles devoted to scientific medicine, Dr. Hurst is a member of the American Heart Association and the American College of Cardiology, and was selected Master of the American College of Physicians. He received the B.S. degree (1941) from the University of Georgia, Atlanta, and the M.D. degree (1944) from the Medical College of Georgia, Augusta, and was a cardiology fellow with Dr. Paul White at Massachusetts General Hospital, Boston.

Part I

How People Learn

Chapter 1

The Learning Process

Some readers may believe that this chapter should not be included in this book. Accordingly, I wish to present a few points in favor of doing so.

The word *learning* is commonly misused. We see signs that identify a "learning center" when in fact the facility provides only a source for information. We observe persons who when exposed to information that is dispensed by lecturers or is discovered on the Internet say they are learning; in reality, they are only registering a few bits of information in the brain. Some people believe that they have learned something when they receive an A in a course whose subject matter they have memorized, only to find out a short while later that they remember very little about it. Although no data are available on the subject, I suspect that the word *learning* is used improperly more than any other word in the English language.

To understand learning it is necessary to define *information*, *memory*, *thinking*, and *learning*. These words, and the mental activity they represent, have been studied by thoughtful individuals for many centuries. More recently, after the development of magnetic resonance imaging (MRI), the mind itself has been studied by psychologists and neuroanatomists. *Mapping the Mind*, a page-turner by Rita Carter, describes the human mind.(1) Her book, which includes photographs of MRI scans taken while the subject's mind is registering images, storing information, and thinking, should be read by all who are interested in the subject.

GENERAL COMMENTS ABOUT THE COMPONENTS OF THE LEARNING PROCESS

Information

Information is discovered by our five senses (2). It should be viewed initially as signals that are momentarily flashed to specific places in the brain. Information gained by visualization is registered in one area of the brain, information gained by hearing in another. The registration of faces is located in one part of the brain, and the registration of abstract objects in a different part. The deflections seen in the electrocardiogram are undoubtedly registered as objects.

Memory

Information that is discovered using our five senses is registered in the brain but it may or may not be stored there. During the first few years of life, few memories are stored, because the brain is not fully developed. Later, the child stores some of the images he or she is exposed to within the family circle. Still later, the child is expected to memorize and store abstract concepts such as the multiplication tables; he or she does so by repeating the tables over and over and over.

When information is registered in the brain, the thinking individual must make a conscious decision regarding the worth of storing the information. If that is not done, the brain will become filled with useless information. If the person decides the information is worth storing, he or she should consciously do one or both of the following things in order to create a reliable memory. *The information being stored must be used frequently or it must be linked to other information already stored in the brain that is used frequently.*(2).

Thinking

Thinking entails the realignment or manipulation of memories.(2,3). Some of the memories may have been stored years earlier, some stored more recently, and some only milliseconds before the active process known as thinking begins. Thinking requires that the person doing it focus his or her mind on the realignment process. In that way the individual is able to give undivided attention to the mental activity that is dominating the moment. When focusing is done well, the person thinking may not hear a telephone ring or hear the voices of someone who addresses him or her. When the rearrangement of memories creates a new perception for the one doing the rearranging the process is known as thinking.

Learning (4)

Suppose a person wishes to learn a foreign language. How will the person determine if he or she has learned the language? One way to find out would be for that individual to visit the country where the language is the native tongue and determine if the natives have trouble understanding him or her. If the individual can communicate easily, it would indicate the person had done enough practice to attain proficiency.

The point of the example just stated is that learning implies that a physical skill, such as swimming, or a mental skill, such as thinking, requires knowledge as to how the skill is performed and then, in addition, requires practice, practice, and more practice, often under supervision, until the person trying to learn the skill is *fluent*.

There is another feature of learning that should be mentioned. Fluency, as described above, indicates that the person has practiced and practiced the task until he or she can perform as an expert performs. Should individuals attain such fluency they will retain a high degree of proficiency even if they do not perform the task for a period of time. Should that occur, individuals who are fluent will be a little slow when they return to the task, but after a short period of time, they will achieve their former competence. On the other hand, individuals who never became fluent in the first place will have to start over after they have been removed from the task for a period of time, because they will perform like a beginner.

Learning is a complex mental task that involves the *registration* of information in the brain, the creation of *memories* by storing the information in the brain, the ability to *recall* the information that is stored, *manipulation or rearrangement of information* in the brain, and the repetition of the physical or mental act until the individual is *fluent*.

HOW TO LEARN TO INTERPRET ELECTROCARDIOGRAMS

Obviously, learning to interpret electrocardiograms must be viewed in the light of the comments made about learning in general.

First of all, the clinician who is trying to learn to interpret electrocardiograms must realize that the goal of the endeavor is to determine the type of heart disease that could cause the electrocardiographic abnormalities. In other words, the electrocardiogram is a diagnostic tool. Competence is determined by how well the "interpreter" can achieve the stated goal.

The waves noted in the electrocardiogram must obviously be observed by the interpreter. They are at that moment viewed as abstract objects. The images of the objects are registered in a special part of the brain. A deliberate decision is then made, which may be right or wrong, about the need to reject or store the images of the objects. The storage of images creates memories that can, when the need arises, be called for active duty. The problem is that the brain has a limited ability to store abstract and poorly understood images. Computers are much better than the brain in accomplishing that act. However, human memories can be enhanced by repeated use of the images and by linking the newly registered information to commonly used information that is already stored in the brain. For one trying to learn to interpret electrocardiograms, it means that the struggling interpreter must inspect numerous electrocardiograms as often as possible and *must link the information that is gathered from each tracing to the commonly used basic principles of electrocardiography, including vector concepts, that are stored in the brain.* This is what this book is about. As experience is gained interpreting more and more electrocardiograms, more and more memories can be stored and, when they are linked to basic principles, not only are they available for recall, they are understood. When this is achieved, the memories can be rearranged or manipulated into new perceptions—a process we call thinking.

In addition, individuals must improve the speed with which they interpret electrocardiograms by making the effort each time they see an electrocardiogram. This, we now know, leads to the fluency that improves the memory of the interpreter.

After all this, the interpreter must correlate the other clinical data with the electrocardiographic data in order to gradually add to his or her list of heart diseases that could cause the electrocardiographic abnormalities.

Persons who try to memorize the shape of electrocardiographic abnormalities but know no basic principles of electrocardiography will fail to learn electrocardiography. Persons

who use basic principles, including vector concepts, to interpret each electrocardiogram will be far more proficient—but
they too will sometimes be bewildered because the heart does
not give up its secrets without a struggle!

A TEST FOR THE READER*

I ask the reader to take the following test (2): Multiply 8 times
6. The answer is easy. Multiple 9 times 6. The answer is easy.
This is because we all memorized the multiplication tables in
the early years of our schooling. Note that the numbers in the
tables we memorized are single digits. Suppose you are asked
to multiply 23 times 10. This too is easy because one of the
double digits is 10. As is obvious, a double digit in which the
second digit is 0 is also used in multiplication without diffi-
culty. Now suppose you are asked to multiply 23 times 9. This
is not as easy as multiplying single digits. When asked to multiply 23 times 58, you resort to a *system of multiplying* that
requires the use of several steps. The point is, memory has its
limitations. Should a person wish to multiply more than single
digits, he or she must have a *system of multiplying*. Without
such a system, an individual would be greatly limited because
there are more numbers beyond the single digits that need to
be multiplied than there are numbers under the number 10.
The same is true for electrocardiography: a person can memorize a few electrocardiographic patterns, but beyond a limited
number he or she needs *a system to interpret the large number
of tracings that lie outside the scope of his or her memory.* The
purpose of this book is to discuss the *system* used to interpret
electrocardiograms.

---

* The concept expressed in the section entitled "A Test for the Reader" is
similar to that expressed by me in reference 2. The text, however, is quite
different.

REFERENCES

1. Carter R. Mapping the Mind. Berkeley: University of California Press, 1998.

2. Hurst JW. Methods used to interpret the 12-lead electrocardiogram: Pattern memorization versus the use of vector concepts. Clin Cardiol 2000;23:4–13.

3. Stead EA Jr. Thinking ward rounds. Medical Times 1967;95: 706–708.

4. Hurst JW. Teaching Medicine: Process, Habits, and Actions. Atlanta: Scholars Press, 1999:22–24.

Part II

Historical Benchmarks and the Naming of the Waves

Chapter 2

The People and the Waves

Almost everyone recognizes the names Babe Ruth, Hank Aaron, Michael Jordan, Bobby Jones, Elvis Presley, George Washington, and Oliver Wendell Holmes Jr. Most of the people who know these names do not plan to participate in the games of baseball, basketball, or golf or intend to become rock music stars, politicians, or judges. People remember the names because they are interested in what those individuals did. On the other hand, trainees in medicine and practicing physicians who record electrocardiograms may know little about the important people who contributed greatly to the development of the procedure and the interpretation of the tracings. This chapter contains a list of a few innovative people who paved the way for the rest of us and includes a brief description of the naming of the waves.

THE PEOPLE

Hundreds of people have contributed to the knowledge of electrocardiography, but the individuals discussed here deserve special recognition because their work formed the basis for this book (see Fig. 2-1).

Augustus D. Waller (1856–1922; see Fig. 2-1A), a British physiologist, used a crude mercury capillary electrometer to record the first human electrocardiogram in 1887 (1,2). He initially labeled the waves V_1 and V_2 because he knew they were ventricular events. As new waves were discovered with the use of improved mercury capillary electrometers, he switched to the letters ABCD.

Willem Einthoven (1860–1927; see Fig. 2-1B), a Dutch physician–scientist, impoved the galvanometer and made many contributions to the field of electrocardiography. He invented the bipolar extremity leads and created Einthoven's law. He named the waves in the electrocardiogram PQRST (1,2).

Sir Thomas Lewis (1881–1945; see Fig. 2-1C), a British physician-scientist, studied the use of the electrocardiogram

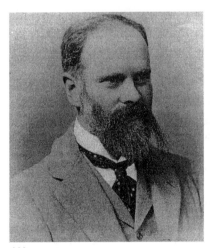

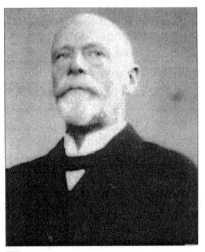

(A)   **(B)**

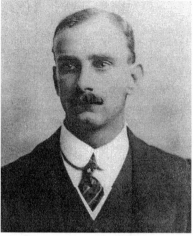

(C)

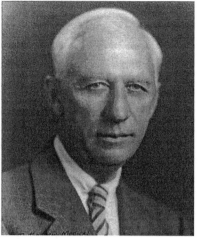

(D)

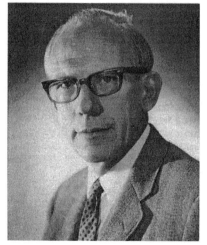

(E)

Figure 2-1 Important contributors to the field of electrocardiography. (All photographs provided by the National Library of Medicine, Bethesda, Maryland.)

A. Augustus D. Waller (1856–1922).

B. Willem Einthoven (1860–1927).

C. Sir Thomas Lewis (1881–1945).

D. Dr. Frank N. Wilson (1890–1952).

E. Dr. Robert P. Grant (1915–1966).

in deciphering arrhythmias and was one of the first electro-
physiologists (2).

Dr. Frank N. Wilson (1890–1952; see Fig. 2-1D), an
American, studied with Lewis. He later worked at the University of Michigan, in Ann Arbor, and became the foremost electrocardiographer in the world. He contributed to the mathematical understanding of the electrocardiogram and invented
the unipolar leads. He stressed the use of basic principles in
the interpretation of electrocardiograms (2,3).

Dr. Robert P. Grant (1915–1966; see Fig. 2-1E), working
at Emory University in Atlanta, Georgia, developed and
taught the use of vector concepts in the interpretation of every
electrocardiogram (2,4). He and Dr. Harvey Estes are responsible for my interest in electrocardiography. In this book, I
have simply expanded the concepts they taught me in 1949/
1950.

THE WAVES

The evolution of the naming of the waves makes interesting
reading. The reader is referred to a recent article for a detailed
account of the subject (1).

The waves seen in most modern electrocardiograms are
shown in Figure 2–2A. Additional waves have been discovered
and they are illustrated in Figures 2-2B through 2-2E. More
waves undoubtedly remain to be discovered.

Figure 2-2   Waves seen in the electrocardiogram.
A. Waves commonly seen in the electrocardiogram (Source: Hurst
JW. *Ventricular Electrocardiography*. New York: Gower Medical
Publishing, 1991:5.7. The author, J.W.H., owns the copyright.)
B. Delta wave.
C. Osborn wave.
D. Epsilon wave.
E. Brugada wave.

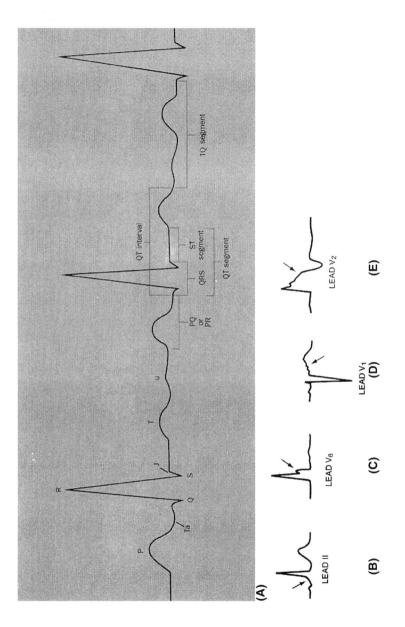

(A)

(B) LEAD II

(C) LEAD V₆

(D) LEAD V₁

(E) LEAD V₂

Einthoven knew the P waves were produced by the electricity created by the atria and realized that the QRS complexes and T waves were produced by the electricity created by the ventricles (1). He originally used the letters ABCD to identify the waves he recorded with a mercury capillary electrometer. The change in lettering was necessary because Einthoven created a mathematical formula that corrected for the inertia in the recording produced by the mercury capillary electrometer. So, I believe (along with Henson) that in order to prevent confusion within a single illustration, he probably labeled the actual curve within the letters ABCD and his mathematically corrected curve, PQRST (1). He probably used the labels PQRST following the scheme of lettering used by Descartes (1). As an afterthought, Einthoven realized that by choosing letters from near the middle of the alphabet, he could add letters before the P and after the T.

When Einthoven began to record electrocardiograms with a galvanometer he continued to label the waves PQRST. Waller, however, did not accept the new lettering (1). The U wave was identified later, when the galvanometer was improved.

The short P-R interval and slurred initial portion of the QRS was noted by *Wilson* (5), *Wedd* (6), and *Hamburger* (7) (see Fig. 2-2B). Over the years, these abnormalities have been noted in retrospect in many published papers and electrocardiograph files but they were not recognized at the time they were recorded. *Wolff, Parkinson,* and *White* identified the relationship of the short P-R interval and slurred initial portion of the QRS complex, to supraventricular tachycardia (8). They did not, however, name the slur of the initial QRS complex a *delta wave. Segers, Lequime,* and *Denolin* used the Greek letter delta to identify the slur in 1944 (9), some 14 years after the paper by Wolff, Parkinson, and White was published. The short P-R interval and slurred initial portion of the QRS complex is now known as preexcitation of the ventricles (see discussion in Chapter 23). It is responsible for episodes of supraventricular tachycardia, including atrial fibrillation.

The hump on the descending portion of the QRS complex

is currently called an *Osborn wave* (see Fig. 2-2C). Although the wave was seen by others, Osborn's excellent description of it has gained widespread attention (10,11). This is now known to be one of the types of post-excitation of the ventricles (see discussion in Chapter 23) and is usually produced by hypothermia.

The wiggles in the ST segment are called *epsilon waves* (see Fig. 2-2D). They were identified by *Fontaine* (1). They are produced by delayed depolarization of a portion of the right ventricle. This is another type of post-excitation of the ventricles (see discussion in Chapter 23) and is seen in patients with right ventricular dysplasia. These patients are subject to episodes of treacherous cardiac arrhythmias. Epsilon waves can also be seen in other conditions, including right ventricular infarction (see Chapter 15).

Noncoronary ST segment displacement due to a genetically determined abnormal action potential curve in the myocytes of a portion of the right ventricle may be seen in the chest leads (V_1-V_3) in patients with right bundle branch block or right ventricular conduction delay. These abnormal waves of repolarization are called *Brugada waves* (1) (see Fig. 2-2E and discussion in Chapter 23). These abnormalities are predictors of serious ventricular arrhythmias and possible death.

REFERENCES

1. Hurst JW. Naming of the waves in the ECG, with a brief account of their genesis. Circulation 1998;98:1937–1942.

2. Hurst JW. Ventricular Electrocardiography. New York: Gower Medical Publishing, 1991:1.1–13.36.

3. Kahn JK, Howell JD. Profile on Frank Norman Wilson. Clin Cardiol 1987;10:616–618.

4. Hurst JW. Profile on Robert Purves Grant. Clin Cardiol 1987; 10:286–287.

5. Wilson FN. A case in which the vagus influenced the form of

the ventricular complex of the electrocrdiogram. Arch Intern Med 1915;16:1008–1027.

6. Wedd AM. Paroxysmal tachycardia; with reference to nomotopic tachycardia and the role of the extrinsic cardiac nerves. Arch Intern Med 1921;27:571–590.

7. Hamburger WW. Bundle-branch block: 4 cases of intraventricular block showing some interesting and unusual clinical features. Med Clin North Am 1929;13:343–362.

8. Wolff L, Parkinson J, White PD. Bundle-branch block with the short P-R interval in healthy young people prone to paroxysmal tachycardia. Am Heart J 1930;5:685–704.

9. Segers PM, Lequime J, Denolin H. L'activation ventriculaire précoc de certains coeurs hyperexcitables: etude de l'onde Δ de l'électrocardiogramme. Cardiologia 1944;8:113–167.

10. Gussak I, Bjerregaard P, Egan TM, Chaitman BR. ECG phenomenon called the J wave: history, pathyophysiology, and clinical significance. J Electrocardiol 1995;28:49–58.

11. Osborn JJ. Experimental hypothermia: respiratory and blood pH changes in relation to cardiac function. Am J Physiol 1953; 175:389–398.

12. Brugada P, Brugada J. Right bundle branch block, persistent ST segment elevation and sudden cardiac death: a distinct clinical and electrocardiographic syndrome: a multicenter report. J Am Coll Cardiol 1992;20:1391–1396.

Part III

Basic Principles of
Electrocardiography

Chapter 3

Memory No. 1: The Use of Vectors to Illustrate the Electrical Forces of the Heart

Every force, be it physical or electrical, has direction and magnitude and can be considered to be a vector. The symbol for a vector is an arrow (see Fig. 3-1). The *length* of the arrow represents the magnitude of the force, and the *inclination* of the arrow represents the direction of the force.

THE USE OF A VECTOR TO ILLUSTRATE A PHYSICAL FORCE

Suppose a truck can pull a log 10 feet every 6 seconds or 100 feet in 1 minute. This event could be diagrammed as shown in Figure 3-2A. Note the direction and length of the arrow.

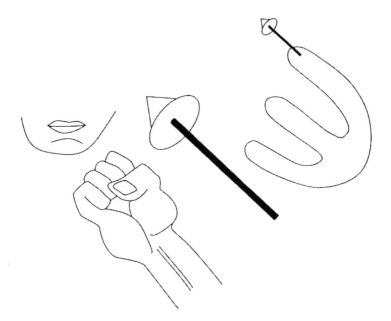

Figure 3-1 The arrow, symbolizing a vector, can be used to represent a physical force (see figure to the left) or an electrical force produced by the heart (see figure to the right).

Figure 3-2 Diagram using vectors to determine and illustrate the direction and distance two trucks can pull a log. *A.* A truck can pull a log 10 feet every 6 seconds or 100 feet in 1 minute. Note that the line illustrating the distance the log is pulled is divided into 10 parts of 10 feet each. *B.* A different trunk can pull a log 10 feet every 3 seconds or 200 feet in 1 minute. Note that the line illustrating the distance the log is pulled is divided into 20 parts of 10 feet each. *C.* Two trucks, functioning simultaneously, pull their usual amount for 1 minute. They pull in different directions because the rough terrain will not allow them to line up in front of the log. *D.* The direction and distance the log will be pulled when the trucks pull simultaneously for 1 minute can be calculated by constructing a parallelogram and drawing a diagonal line as shown above. There are about 28 units in the line representing the diagonal. The log would be moved approximately 280 feet in the direction shown by the diagonal line.

A.

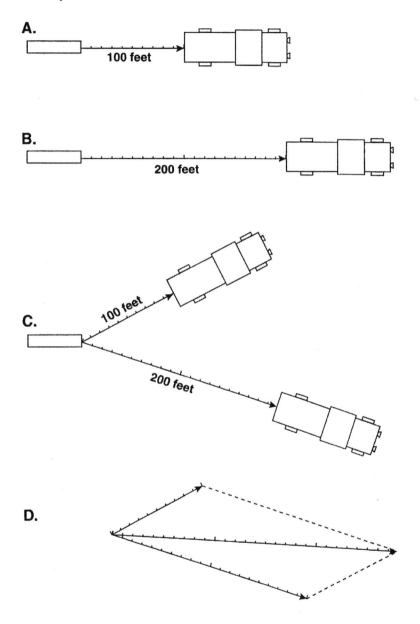

100 feet

B.

200 feet

C.

100 feet

200 feet

D.

Note also that the distance the truck pulls the log in 1 minute is divided into 10 units in which each unit is equal to 10 feet. Now suppose another truck can pull the same log 10 feet every 3 seconds or 200 feet in a minute. The same units of measurement are used in this diagram as were used in Figure 3-2A. This event could be diagrammed as shown in Figure 3-2B. Now imagine that both of the trucks pulled on the same log for one minute but that rocky terrain prevented each of them from locating directly in front of the log, as shown in Figure 3-2C. The two trucks, pulling simultaneously, would drag the log approximately 280 feet in 1 minute and the log would be pulled in the direction shown by the arrow in Figure 3-2D. This figure illustrates how vectors are added together. The direction and distance the log was pulled is illustrated by the diagonal line produced by constructing a parallelogram as shown in Figure 3-2D, in which the vectors produced by the two trucks make up two sides of the figure.

THE USE OF VECTORS TO ILLUSTRATE
THE ELECTRICAL FORCES OF THE HEART

The electrical forces of the heart can also be represented as vectors that are illustrated by arrows. Each minute portion of the atrial and ventricular myocardium produces a small amount of electrical force that is directed up or down, to the right or left; and because the heart is a three-dimensional structure, the electrical forces are also directed anteriorly or posteriorly.

The spatially oriented electrical forces generated by the heart occur in a sequence; they do not occur simultaneously. The shape and size of the P waves, QRS complexes, S-T segments, and T waves seen in the electrocardiogram are determined by the direction and magnitude of the spatially oriented electrical forces that occur in a sequence and the location of the measuring electrodes that are used to record them.

When the electrical forces generated by the heart are represented by spatially oriented vectors that are *visualized and measured*, one is approaching a scientific method of analysis. The method of achieving this desirable goal is discussed in the subsequent pages of this book.

Chapter 4

Memory No. 2: The Electrical Activity of a Single Isolated Myocyte

The myocardium of the atria and ventricles is made of millions of cells called myocytes. They generate the electrical activity that produces the waves that are recorded in the surface electrocardiogram. The electrical stimulus, in turn, causes the myocytes to contract. It should be emphasized, however, that the flow of electrons that produces the electricity is not the same process as the ionic reaction that causes the myocytes to contract.

The *resting* myocardial cell produces no electrical activity. Such a cell is illustrated in Figure 4-1A. Note that there are negative charges inside the cell that are balanced by positive charges on the outside of the cellular membrane. Such a cell is also said to be *polarized* because both the negative and positive charges are intact and balanced. When the cell is

RIGHT   LEFT

A. Polarized myocyte

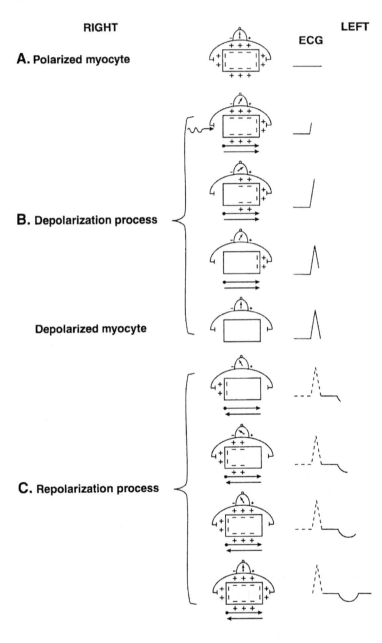

B. Depolarization process

Depolarized myocyte

C. Repolarization process

Figure 4-1 A simplified view of the depolarization and repolarization of a single myocyte. This teaching diagram is an oversimplification of the complex process known as depolarization and repolarization. The diagram was created after studying the works of Barker (1) and Burch and Winsor (2). *A.* A single myocyte that is polarized. Note that the negative electrical charges located inside the cell are balanced by positive changes located on the cell membrane. The simple measuring device is registering zero. Note that the electrode on the right side of the cell (the reader's left side) is hooked to the negative pole of the measuring device and that the electrode on the left side of the cell (the reader's right side) is hooked to the positive pole of the measuring device. Remember, the myocyte is a three-dimensional structure. *B.* The four diagrams represent the depolarization process. Note the large wavy arrow on the right (the reader's left side) in the top panel. It represents the electrical stimulus that is provided by the electrical activity that is transmitted by the conduction system of the heart. When the cell is electrically stimulated, it begins to lose its electrical changes in a sequence that is illustrated in the next three panels. It is important to understand the meaning of the two long arrows located beneath the myocyte. The top arrow •→ indicates the direction of the depolarization *process* and is directed from right to left (the reader's left to right side). The lower arrow → implies that the *electrical force* produced by the depolarization process is also directed from right to left (the reader's left to right). Note how the small arrow in the measuring device moves to its maximum in the second panel and back to 0 when the cell is completely depolarized as shown in the lower panel. The QRS complex is upright (positive) because the depolarization process is directed toward the positive pole of the measuring device. *C.* These four panels illustrate the repolarization process. The top panel shows the electrical charges being restored on the right side (the reader's left side) of the myocyte. Assuming that each part of the cell membrane repolarizes following the same time interval after depolarization, the electrical charges will be restored on the right side (the reader's left side) of the cell where they were initially lost. The two arrows shown at the lower part of each of the three panels are very important. The upper arrow •→ illustrates the direction of the repolarization *process.* The lower arrow ← indicates the direction of the *electrical force* produced by the repolarization process. Note that the direction of the *repolarization process* is opposite to the direction of the *electrical force* it produces. Accordingly, the T wave is negative or inverted and is directed opposite to the QRS complex. As discussed later, the concept expressed here forms the conceptual basis for understanding normal and abnormal QRS and T waves.

stimulated on the right side (the reader's left side), it sets in motion the loss of the electrical charges (see Fig. 4-1B). The process of losing electrical charges is called *depolarization*. When the cell has lost all of its charges it is called a *depolarized* or *excited* cell (see lower illustration in Fig. 4-1B). After a brief delay the electrical charges begin to reappear on the cell. They reappear first on the right side (the reader's left side) of the cell, where they were initially lost. This process is called *repolarization* and, assuming there is an equal delay throughout the cell between the time the electrical charges were lost to the time they were restored, the repolarization process will follow the same path taken by depolarization (see Fig. 4-1C). That is to say, under the circumstances depicted above, *the direction of the depolarization process predetermines the direction of repolarization process.*

Thus far we have looked only at a single myocardial cell, but the heart is composed of millions of cells. The myocardial cells produce electrical forces (vectors) that are directed up or down, right or left, and anteriorly or posteriorly. As will be discussed, there is an orderly sequence to the generation of electrical forces by the heart. The shape of the P, QRS, S-T, T, and U waves in the electrocardiogram would not exist if all of the cells in the heart depolarized simultaneously and then repolarized simultaneously. The waves are produced because the numerous instantaneous electrical forces that are produced by the depolarization and repolarization of the normal and abnormal atrial and ventricular myocytes have different sizes, are directed in different directions, and are not produced simultaneously.

REFERENCES

1. Barker JM. *The Unipolar Electrocardiogram: A Clinical Interpretation*. New York: Appleton-Century-Crofts, Inc., 1952: 37–76.

2. Burch G, Winsor T. *A Primer of Electrocardiography*. Philadelphia: Lea & Febiger, 1947:26–31 (first printed 1945).

Chapter 5

Memory No. 3: The Volume Conductor and the Spread of Electrical Activity to the Body Surface

THE BODY AS A VOLUME CONDUCTOR

The routine electrocardiogram is recorded by placing electrodes on the body surface and attaching them by wires to the electrocardiograph machine. A recording is possible because the electricity generated by the heart spreads through the tissues of the body to reach the skin. The tissues are viewed collectively as a *volume conductor* (1). Tissues such as the lungs, bones, muscles, and skin offer different resistances to the transmission of the electrical activity generated by the heart and, because of this, the body is not considered to be a homogeneous conductor of electricity. However, for practical clinical purposes, we assume that the tissues of the body are fairly good conductors of electrical activity.

THE ELECTRICAL FIELD

It should be obvious: an *electrical field* produced by an electrical force originating in the heart will spread inferiorly, superiorly, to the right or left, and anteriorly and posteriorly to reach the body surface. It is useful to remember that a live electric wire in a swimming pool will create electrical activity throughout the pool.

The Graphic Representation of the Three Components of an Electrical Field

An electrical force generated by the heart creates an electrical field that has the characteristics that are shown graphically in Figure 5-1. The electrical force, which is represented as a

---

Figure 5-1   The electrical field created by an electrical force. *A.* A frontal view of an electrical field. The origin of the electrical force is located at the center of the cylinder. Note the zero potential plane that separates the positive and negative halves of he electrical field. The zero potential plane is perpendicular to the direction of electrical force and, when it extends to the body surface, it becomes the transitional pathway. The rings represent lines of equipotentiality. For simplicity, only three rings are shown. This schematic illustration is not intended to show all the details of an electrical field. (*Source*: Hurst JW, Woodson GC Jr. *Atlas of Spatial Vector Electrocardiography*. New York: The Blakiston Company, Inc, 1952:8. The author, J.W.H., owns the copyright.) *B.*   An electrical field in three-dimensional space. The lines of equipotential are illustrated as spheres (or shells). For simplicity, only three shells are shown. The zero potential plane is perpendicular to the direction of electrical force, and when it extends to the body surface, it becomes the transitional pathway. This simple diagram is not intended to represent all that is known about an electrical field. (*Source*: Hurst JW, Woodson GC Jr. *Atlas of Spatial Vector Electrocardiography*. New York: The Blakiston Company, Inc, 1952:8. The author, J.W.H., owns the copyright.)

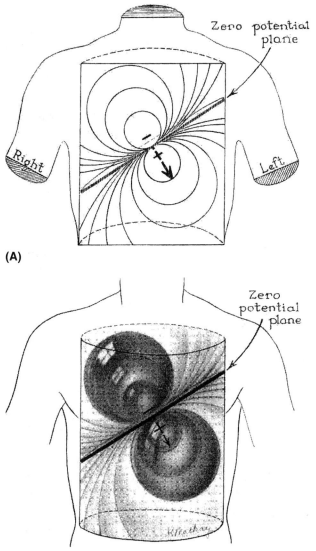

(A)

(B)

vector, should be assumed to *originate in the "center" of the heart, which is near the "center" of the chest.* As will become apparent later, this assumption is a reasonable one to make. The *zero potential plane* is a three-dimensional structure that is located at the origin of the electrical force; it is perpendicular to the direction of the vector that represents the direction of the electrical force. It divides the entire body into electrically negative and positive "halves." The zero potential plane extends to the body surface, where it produces the *transitional pathway* that separates an area of negativity from an area of positivity on the body surface.

Isopotential Spheres or Shells

The electrical field produced by an electrical force is made up of a series of larger and larger isopotential spheres (or shells). This means that the electrical potential will be the same wherever it is measured within the spheres or shells. The isopotential spheres (or shells) become larger and larger the greater the distance they are from the origin of the electrical forces that produces them. The *frontal plane view* of an electrical field is shown in Figure 5-1A. Note the direction of the electrical force, the zero potential plane, and the isopotential lines that are shown as rings. Note how the rings become larger and larger. In order to simplify the concept, the chest itself is shown as a cylinder. The *spatial view* of the electrical field is shown in Figure 5-1B. The isopotential lines are not rings; they are spheres (or shells). Note the location of the *zero potential plane* that is perpendicular to the electrical force. Note also that it extends to the body surface, where it becomes the *transitional pathway* that divides the body into positive and negative regions.

Another important basic principle is germane to this particular discussion: *The amount of electrical potential varies inversely with the square of the distance.* This is why the isopotential spheres become larger and larger. As discussed later, this is the basis for Einthoven's law and is why we can use the deflections recorded in the extremity leads and, to some degree, the deflection recorded in the chest leads to determine the spatial direction of electrical forces.

As the contents of this book unfold, the electrical forces of the heart will be considered to be vectors, and arrows will be used to illustrate them.

Having read this chapter, the reader should now look more carefully at the arrows used to illustrate electrical forces (see Fig. 5-2). The *length of the arrow signifies the magnitude*, or size, of the electrical force it represents. The *inclination of the arrow* indicates the direction of the electrical force. The arrowhead indicates the *polarity* of the electrical force. That is, when the vector is directed toward the positive electrode of the measuring device, an upright or positive recording will be produced. When the vector is directed away from the positive

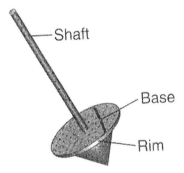

Figure 5-2   An arrow (the symbol for a vector) has three parts: the shaft, the base of the arrowhead, and the rim of the arrowhead. The base of the arrowhead represents the zero potential plane. The rim of the arrowhead represents the transitional pathway. The length of the shaft represents the magnitude of the electrical force. The inclination of the arrow represents the orientation of the electrical force in space. The arrowhead indicates the polarity (the sense) of the force, which, taken along with its inclination, indicates the direction of the force. (*Source*: Hurst JW. *Cardiovascular Diagnosis: The Initial Examination.* St. Louis: Mosby, 1993:199. The author, J.W.H., owns the copyright.)

electrode of the measuring device, a downward or negative re-cording will be produced. *The base of the arrow represents the zero potential plane of an electrical force and the rim of the arrow represents the transitional pathway of the electrical force* (see Fig. 5-2).

Chapter 6

Memory No. 4: The Anatomy of the Heart Chambers and Conduction System

A series of vectors can be used to illustrate the directions and sizes of the electrical forces produced by the heart because all of the myocytes do not depolarize and repolarize simultaneously. If they did, they would produce a recording that consisted of spikes only; there would be no contour or shape to the QRS complexes and T waves. This leads one to conclude that the *location of the myocardial cells that cluster together to make the four chambers of the heart, as well as the sequence in which the myocytes are stimulated electrically, are of paramount importance.* Accordingly, this chapter deals with the location and anatomic features of the heart chambers and conduction system because they play a major role in determining the directions and sizes of the electrical forces that create the deflections seen in the electrocardiogram.

THE LOCATION AND ANATOMIC FEATURES
OF THE HEART CHAMBERS

The anatomic information about the heart chambers needed to interpret electrocardiograms is shown in Figure 6-1. The magnetic resonance images of the chest that are shown in the figure were made of a house officer in normal health.

The *frontal view* shown in Figure 6-1A reveals that the *anatomic axis* of the *left ventricle* of the adult is directed to the left and inferiorly. As will be discussed later, the direction of the electrical axis of the heart is different from the direction of the anatomic axis of the heart. The *right atrium* produces the right lateral portion of the heart. The *right ventricle* is not seen, because it is an anterior structure. It lies to the right of the left ventricle, but it is located anteriorly. The *left atrium* cannot be seen but it is located posteriorly in the middle of the cardiac silhouette just beneath the bifurcation of the trachea into the bronchi (1).

The *lateral view* shown in Figure 6-1B reveals that the *anatomic axis* of the left ventricle is directed anteriorly and inferiorly. The anterior direction of the anatomic axis of the left ventricle is not generally appreciated. The right ventricle can be seen anteriorly (1).

The *transverse views* shown in Figure 6-1C, reveal that the *anatomic axis of the left ventricle* is directed to the left and anteriorly. The *right ventricle* is seen anteriorly. The *left atrium* is not located on the left as the name implies; it is located posteriorly between the vertebrae and the remainder of the heart. The *right atrium* is located to the right of, and anterior to, the left atrium (1).

If one wishes to examine an organ, it is essential to know where the organ is located in the body. The diagrams shown in Figure 6-1 illustrate the location of the chambers of the heart when the subject is lying down. The location of the heart changes slightly when the patient stands or is seated. This information is needed not only to interpret electrocardiograms but also to interpret the pulsations that are palpated on the anterior and lateral portion of the chest and to interpret a chest x-ray film.

Additional information is provided in the diagram shown in Figure 6-2. This figure shows other important anatomic structures, including the location of the coronary arteries, as they are seen in the frontal view.

The image of the anatomy of the heart shown in Figures 6-1 and 6-2 must be stored in the working memory bank of the brain, for they must be recalled whenever each electrocardiogram is interpreted.

THE LOCATION AND ANATOMIC FEATURES OF THE CONDUCTION SYSTEM

The *sinus node* is located where the superior vena cava enters the right atrium (see Fig. 6-3A). This remarkable structure is capable of *spontaneous depolarization* 60 to 80 times each minute unless it becomes "sick" or some other heart rhythm becomes dominant.

The electrical activity created by the sinus node stimulates the *right atrial myocytes* to depolarize. The wave of depolarization spreads over the atrial myocytes like the fall of a series of dominoes that are lined up in a row. There is an argument regarding the presence or absence of specialized cells in the atria that conduct electrical activity as the bundle branches do in the ventricles. While the argument is not settled, one can state with certainty that there are several *preferential pathways* that seem to guide the direction of the electrical activity within the right and left atrial walls (see Fig. 6-3A).

The wave of depolarization spreads initially into the right atrium and produces the first half of the P wave. The wave of depolarization then spreads into the left atrium and produces the second half of the P wave. The individual who uses images to think can visualize the anatomic location of the right atrium and the wave of depolarization of the right atrium when he or

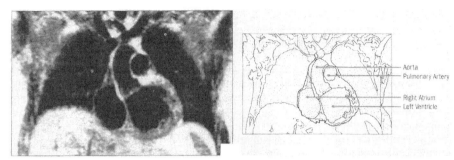

(A)

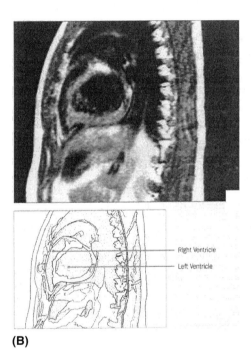

(B)

Figure 6-1 The anatomy of the heart. The house officer was lying down when these magnetic resonance images were made of his heart. *A.* Frontal view. *B.* Saggital view. *C* and *D.* Two different transverse views. (*Source*: Hurst JW: *Ventricular Electrocardiography*. New York: Gower Medical Publishing, 1991:4.6 and 4.7. The author, J.W.H., owns the copyright.)

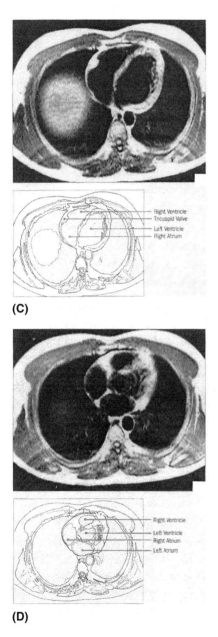

(C)

(D)

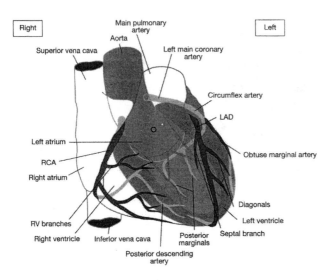

Figure 6-2 The anatomy of the heart. This frontal view of the heart shows the location of the right atrium, left atrium, the aortic valve, and the coronary arteries. RCA = right coronary artery. RV branches = right ventricular banches of the coronary artery. The posterior descending coronary artery is a branch off the right coronary artery. LAD = left anterior descending coronary artery. The diagonals are branches off the left anterior descending coronary artery, and the marginals are branches off the circumflex coronary artery. The artist has made the anterior portion of the arteries dark gray and the posterior portion of the arteries a lighter shade of gray. (Source: Hurst JW. Methods used to interpret the 12-lead electrocardiogram: Pattern memorization versus the use of vector concepts. *Clinical Cardiology* 2000;23:4–13. Used with permission.)

she views the first half of the P waves and can visualize the anatomic location of the left atrium and the wave of depolarization of the left atrium when he or she views the second half of the P waves.

The *atrioventricular node* is located in the lower part of the right atrium (Fig. 6-3A). The conduction of electricity is slowed by this structure.

The *bundle of His* forms the specialized conduction tissue that connects the A-V node with the conduction system located within the ventricles (Fig. 6-3A).

It has been customary to refer to the *right and left bundles* of the conduction system that lie within the ventricles. I believe the use of the words *left bundle* are inappropriate because they lead individuals to think in terms of a rope-like structure. Accordingly, I recommend use of the words *left ventricular conduction system* instead of left bundle. A glance at Figure 6-3B belies the view that it is a bundle; the left ventricular conduction system is a fan-like structure. I have no objections to calling the *right bundle* a bundle because it looks like a rope (Fig. 6-3C). Regardless of the names, the electrical activity is transmitted with lightning speed to the myocytes where it is again slowed.

The *left conduction system* is complex and, as emphasized above, is not a bundle; it is a fan (Fig 6-3B). In 1906, Tawara called it tripartate because there are three parts to the fan, which is espaliered on the endocardial surface of the interventricular septum within the left ventricle (2). Tawara's remarkable research is worth reviewing although it was published almost 100 years ago. He discovered that one branch off the fan passed down the anterior portion of the interventricular system and curved anteriorly, superiorly, and leftward (Fig. 6-3D). This branch is now called the *left anterior-superior division of the left conduction system*. He discovered that another branch of the left conduction system was directed inferiorly and posteriorly (Fig. 6-3D). This branch is now called the *left posterior-inferior division* of the left conduction system. The third part of the broad fan-like structure is located in between the two branches described above. We know that the middle part of the septum is depolarized initially, producing the first part of the QRS complex (3). Perhaps the early branches to the *interventricular septum* originate from the broad middle part of the structure (see Fig. 6-3D).

The branches of the left conduction system transmit elec-

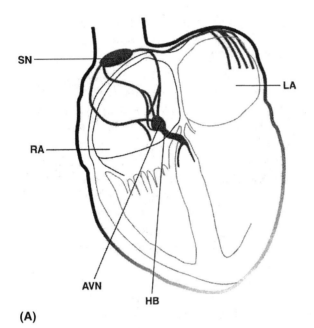

(A)

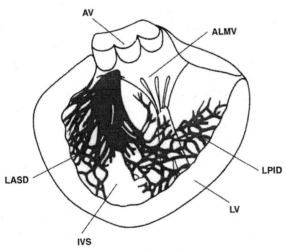

(B)

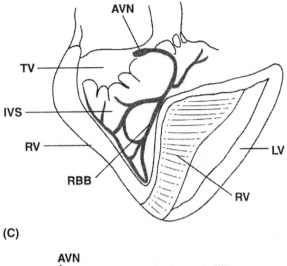

(C)

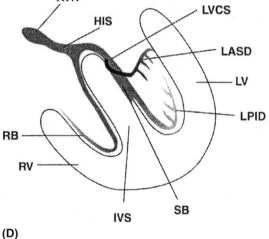

(D)

Figure 6-3 The location and anatomic features of the conduction system. *A. The atrial conduction system showing the location of the sinus node (SN), the preferential conduction pathways, the atrioventricular node (AVN), and His bundle (HB). B.* The left ventricular conduction system (formerly called the left bundle). The diagram is the atrist's rendition of Tawara's photograph of the fan-like structure currently referred to as the left ventricular conduction system. The left ventricle has been pulled to the side, showing that the conduction system is initially espaliered on the endocardial surface of the septum. It produces the left anterior superior division (LASD)

trical stimuli to the myocytes located in the septum, and the anterior, superior, inferior, and posterior parts of the left ventricle.

The right conduction system looks more like a rope, and the words *right bundle* are more appropriately used to describe it (Fig. 6-3D). The right bundle passes down the right ventricular side of the interventricular septum and curves to

---

Figure 6-3 continued   and the left posterior inferior division (LPID) of the left ventricular conduction system. ALMV = anterior leaf of the mitral valve. AV = aortic valve. LV = left ventricle. IVS = interventricular septum. (*Source*: S. Tawara's monograph, Das Reizleitungssystem des Säugetierherzens—Eine anatomisch–histologische Studie über das Atrioventrikular-bündel und die Purkinjeschen Fäden, published in 1906 from Gustav Fischer Verlag in Jena.) *C.*The right bundle branch. The diagram is the artist's rendition of Tawara's photograph of the right bundle branch. AVN = atrioventricular node. TV = tricuspid valve. IVS = interventricular septum. RV = right ventricle. RBB = right bundle branch. LV = left ventricle. The right ventricle has been pulled aside to reveal the interventricular septum from the right side. (*Source*: S. Tawara's monograph, Das Reizleitungssystem des Säugetierherzens—Eine anatomisch–histologische Studie über das Atrioventrikular-bündel und die Purkinjeschen Fäden, published in 1906 from Gustav Fischer Verlag in Jena.) *D.* Diagram of ventricular conduction system. This diagram illustrates the parts of the conduction system that are currently used in the interpretation of electrocardiograms. As can be seen by comparing this diagram wih figures 6–3B and 6–3C, the illustration is a simplification of the actual conduction system. In addition, the physical features of the conduction system vary from person to person. AVN = atrioventricular node. HIS = His bundle. RB = right bundle. RV = right ventricle. IVS = interventricular septum. SB = septal branch. LPID = left posterior inferior division. LV = left ventricle. LASD = left anterior superior division. LVCS=left ventricular conduction system. As illustrated, the black part of the conduction system is located anteriorly and the white part is located posteriorly.

supply the electrical stimulus to the inferior, anterior, and superior portion of the right ventricle.

The left and right conduction systems are completed when the small branches of the conduction system make contact with the myocytes. The final branches of the conduction system are called *Purkinje fibers*. The electricity passes rapidly down the left and right conduction systems, including the Purkinje fibers, and stimulate the myocytes, where the conduction is again slowed. The surface electrocardiogram does not record the electrical activity of the conduction system; the waves in the surface electrocardiogram are made by the electrical forces produced by the atrial and ventricular myocytes. As stated earlier, some of the myocytes are stimulated simultaneously; many of them are stimulated earlier or later than others. This is why there is a contour to the QRS complexes and T waves.

HOW THIS INFORMATION IS USED IN A THOUGHT PROCESS

As a preview to the more detailed discussion presented subsequently, it may be useful to illustrate how some of the information that has been presented thus far is used in a thought process.

The arrows shown in Figure 6-4A symbolize the direction of the electrical forces produced during the first, second, and third parts of the QRS complex. Arrow 1 represents the mean direction of electrical forces produced by early depolarization of the ventricles. Arrow 2 represents the mean direction of the electrical forces produced by depolarization of the ventricles occurring during the next few milliseconds. Arrow 3 represents the electrical forces that are produced by the ventricular myocytes that are depolarized last. The myocytes that are stimulated last are activated almost simultaneously by the left anterior superior division branch and the left posterior in-

(A)

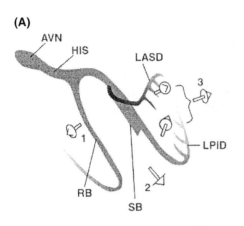

(B)

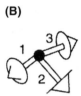

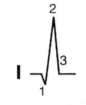

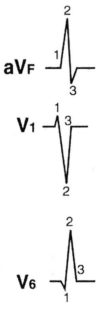

ferior division branch of the left ventricular conduction system. They are shown in Figure 6-4A as two unlabeled arrows. The vector sum of these two electrical forces produce arrow 3, which represents the mean direction of the last electrical forces produced by the depolarization process in the ventricles.

The three labeled arrows shown in Figure 6-4A are assumed to originate from a common point in the center of the heart (Fig. 6–4B). The three spatially oriented arrows, which represent three electrical forces, project onto the measuring system to produce the QRS deflections shown on the right of Figure 6-4B. The numbers on the deflection correspond with the vectors that are identified with similar numbers.

It should be obvious that when an interpreter inspects the deflections of an electrocardiogram and determines the spatial direction of the electrical forces that produce them, he or she should be able to deduce the appropriate anatomic part of the heart that is responsible for them. This overview is provided here in an effort to prepare the reader for a more de-

---

Figure 6-4   The electrical forces produced by the depolarization of certain parts of the heart. *A*. Arrow 1 illustrates the spatial orientation of the electrical forces produced during the early part of depolarization of the ventricles. Arrow 2 illustrates the spatial orientation of the mean electrical forces produced during the next few milliseconds of depolarization of the ventricles. Arrow 3 is produced by the vector sum of the two unlabeled arrows that represent the mean direction of the depolarization of the left ventricular myocytes that are stimulated almost simultaneously by the left anterior superior division and left posterior inferior division of the left ventricular conduction system. *B*. The three labeled arrows are assumed to originate from a common point and project onto the measuring system to create different shapes of QRS complexes (see text). This illustration presents a crude general view about the depolarization of the ventricles; how the electrical forces are projected onto the measuring system (leads); and how an interpreter can visualize the approximate anatomic parts of the ventricles that produce the electrical forces. The details of this thought process are discussed in Chapters 7 and 8.

Chapter 7

Memory No. 5: Depolarization and Repolarization of the Atria and Ventricles; the S-T Segment; and U, Delta, Osborn, Epsilon, and Brugada Waves

THE DEPOLARIZATION AND REPOLARIZATION OF THE ATRIA

Depolarization of the Atria and the Production of P Waves

The first half of the P wave is produced by depolarization of the right atrium (see Fig. 7-1A). The second half of the P wave is produced by depolarization of the left atrium (see Fig. 7-1B).

The normal mean P vector is directed at about 45° to 60° in the frontal plane and is parallel with or slightly anterior to the frontal plane (see Fig. 7-1C). A vector representing the first half of the P wave is normally directed at 45° to 60° in

Right　　　　　　　　　　　　　　　　　　**Left**

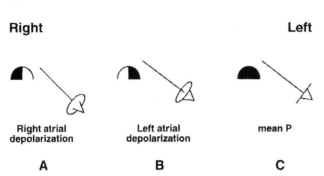

Right atrial　　　Left atrial　　　mean P
depolarization　　depolarization

A　　　　　　　　　B　　　　　　　　C

Figure 7-1 The creation of the P waves. *A*. The first half of the P wave is produced by depolarization of the right atrium. The vector representing this event is directed inferiorly, to the left and slightly anteriorly. *B*. The second half of the P wave is produced by depolarization of the left ~~ventricle~~. The vector representing this event is directed to the left, inferiorly, and slightly posteriorly. *C*. The mean of all of the electrical forces that produce the P wave. The mean P vector is usually directed from 45° to 60° in the frontal plane and about 10° posterior or parallel with the frontal plane.

the frontal plane and about 10° anteriorly. A vector representing the second half of the P wave is normally directed at 45° to 60° in the frontal plane and about 10° posteriorly. A right atrial abnormality usually signifies an abnormality of the right ventricle or tricuspid valve and a left atrial abnormality usually signifies an abnormality of the left ventricle or mitral valve.

Repolarization of the Atria and the Production of the Ta Wave

The atria are relatively thin walled and the pressure within them is low compared to the thick-walled ventricles, within which the pressure is high. Accordingly, the direction of the repolarization process of the atrial myocytes is not influenced by wall thickness and transmyocardial pressure gradient as the repolarization process is in the ventricles. Therefore, the repolarization process follows in the wake of depolarization process and produces electrical forces that are directed opposite to those produced by depolarization. This electrical activity is similar to that occurring in the isolated cell shown in Figure 4.1. The wave of repolarization in the atria is called the Ta wave. The directions of the electrical forces that produce the T of the P are diagrammed in Figure 7-2A. The Ta wave is shown in the deflections illustated in Figure 7-2B. When the P-Q interval is long, the Ta wave may occasionally be seen normally during that segment. When the P-Q interval is short, the Ta wave may occasionally be responsible for the slight depression of the S-T segment of the electrocardiogram.

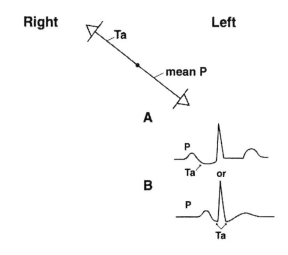

Figure 7-2 The repolarization of the atria (Ta). *A.* The walls of the atrial are thin and the atrial pressure is low compared to that of the ventricles. A mean vector representing the T of the P is directed opposite to the mean vector representing the P wave. *B.* The T of the P (Ta wave) is only occasionally seen. It may produce displacement of the P-Q segment as shown in the two illustrations. The upper illustration shows a depressed P-Q segment when the P-Q interval is long, and the lower illustration shows a depressed P-Q segment and a slightly depressed S-T segment when the P-Q interval is short. An abnormal Ta wave may occur in patients with pericarditis.

DEPOLARIZATION AND REPOLARIZATION
OF THE VENTRICLES

Depolarization of the Ventricles and the
Production of the QRS Complex

Many investigators have studied the sequence of depolarization of the ventricles. Durrer reported his studies on the subject in 1968 (1). These are summarized as follows and are illustrated in Figure 7-3. *Note that the depolarization process of the ventricles is directed predominately from the endocardium to the epicardium.* The illustration and its legend should be studied carefully. The gray portion signifies that the myocytes are polarized. The black area indicates the area of the heart that is undergoing depolarization. The white areas of the heart indicate the areas of the heart that are depolarized and waiting for the repolarization process to begin.

The left inner surface of the *middle part* of the interventricular septum is depolarized initially. This creates the deflection noted in the first 0.01 second of the QRS complex. This can be represented as a mean vector (see Fig. 7-3A). Remember, the septum is not a separate structure; it is simply the portion of the adult's left ventricle that is located anteriorly that separates the left ventricle from the right ventricle. Formerly, most clinicians believed that the upper part of the left side of the septum was the first part of the ventricles to depolarize. Durrer corrected that belief when he discovered that the middle portion of the septum depolarizes first (1). It is noteworthy, however, that the area of the septum that does depolarize initially is rather large. As shown in Figure 7-3A, it creates an electrical force that is usually directed slightly to the right and anteriorly.

During the next 0.02 to 0.03 second (at 0.03 to 0.04 second) of the QRS complex, the endocardial surfaces of both the right and left ventricles are depolarized. This produces electrical forces that can be represented by a vector (see Fig. 7-3B) directed to the left and almost parallel with the frontal plane.

During the next 0.02 to 0.04 second (at about 0.05 to 0.08 second) of the QRS complex, the depolarization process com-

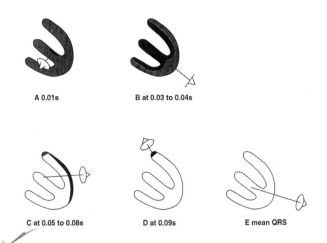

A 0.01s

B at 0.03 to 0.04s

C at 0.05 to 0.08s

D at 0.09s

E mean QRS

Figure 7-3 The sequence of depolarization of the ventricles. *A*. Depolarization of the left middle portion of the septum occurs during the initial 0.01 second of the QRS complex. The black area of the ventricles indicates the portion of the heart that is in the process of being depolarized. The gray areas of the ventricles indicate myocardium that is polarized and waiting to be stimulated. *B*. Depolarization of the endocardial area of both ventricles at 0.03 to 0.04 second of the QRS complex. The black area of the ventricles indicates the portion of the heart that is in the process of being depolarized. The gray areas of the ventricles indicate myocardium that is polarized and waiting to be stimulated. *C*. Depolarization of the lateral portion of the left ventricle at 0.05 to 0.08 second of the QRS complex. The black area of the ventricles indicates the portion of the heart that is in the process of being depolarized. The white area of the ventricles indicates the portion of the heart that has already depolarized and is waiting to be repolarized. The small gray area of the heart is polarized and waiting to be depolarized. *D*. Depolarization of the superior portion of the left ventricle at 0.09 second of the QRS complex. The black area of the ventricles indicates the portion of the heart that is in the process of being depolarized. The white area of the ventricles indicates the portion of the heart that has already depolarized and is waiting to be repolarized. *E*. The normal mean QRS vector of the adult is usually directed to the left, inferiorly and posteriorly. Note that the entire heart is white, indicating that depolarization has been completed. The heart is waiting for the repolarization process to commence.

pletes its spread through the entire right ventricle and most of the left ventricle. This activity leaves a large portion of the heart depolarized. This is shown in white in Figure 7-3C. The part of the left ventricle that is undergoing depolarization is shown in black in figure 7–3C. The electrical forces produced by the depolarization of this area of the left ventricle may be directed to the left and posteriorly. The small gray area of the left ventricle is polarized; it is waiting to undergo depolarization.

During the last 0.01 second (at 0.08 to 0.09 second), the wave of depolarization completes its spread through the left ventricle. This produces the terminal deflection of the QRS complex. The portion of the heart that has already depolarized is shown in white. The last part of the heart to depolarize is shown in black. Note that it is located superiorly in the left ventricle (see Fig. 7-3D). Remember, the base of the heart is located posterior to the apex of the heart. Accordingly, the vector representing these electrical forces is directed posteriorly. The electrical force produced by the depolarization of this portion of the left ventricle may be directed to the right or left depending on the location of the left ventricle in the chest.

The mean direction of the depolarization process described above will be the sum of the vectors representing the depolarization of each part of the ventricles (see Fig. 7-3E). The normal mean QRS vector in the adult is usually directed to the left, inferiorly, and posteriorly, whereas the anatomic axis of the heart is directed to the left, inferiorly, and anteriorly. The direction of the mean QRS vector does not parellel the direction of the anatomic axis because the left posterior-inferior division of the left ventricular conduction system transmits the electrical stimulus to the myocytes located in the posterior portion of the left ventricle.

The shape of the QRS complex is determined by the direction and size of the electrical forces produced by the depolarization process, the thickness of the ventricular muscle, and the normalcy of the myocytes. The discussion above holds for the newborn, adolescent, and adult as far as the *sequence* of depolarization is concerned. One must remember, however, that the *right ventricle in the newborn is as thick or thicker than the left ventricle* and that the septum tends to conform to the shape of the right ventricle. These differences from adult anatomy influence the direction of the depolarization process in the infant and adolescent.

The mean QRS vector may become *abnormally large* due to left or right ventricular hypertrophy or abnormally small due to pericardial effusion or myocardial disease. The *duration* of the QRS complex and the direction of the mean QRS vector becomes abnormal when there is left or right ventricular conduction system disease secondary to certain disease processes.

The direction and size of the initial 0.03 to 0.04 second of the QRS complex is altered with myocardial infarction, and the terminal 0.03 to 0.04 second of the QRS cinokex is altered when there is left or right conduction system block.

Repolarization of the Ventricles and the Production of the T Wave

The repolarization of the ventricles produces the T waves in the electrocardiogram. If all physiologic conditions remained the same during repolarization as they were during depolarization of the ventricles, the repolarization process would proceed from the endocardium to epicardium like the depolarization process. Should this be the case, the repolarization process would follow the path of the depolarization and the T forces would be opposite to that of the QRS forces (see Figure 7-4C). This would be similar to the repolarization of the single myocyte shown in Figure 4-1. However, this is not the case; the physiological environment that is present when the T wave is written is different from the physiological environment that is present when the QRS complex is produced. The depolarization of the ventricles, which is directed predominately from endocardium to epicardium, produces mechanical contraction that creates the pressure within the left and right ventricles. On the other hand, the repolarization process that produces the T wave is produced at the end of mechanical systole of the

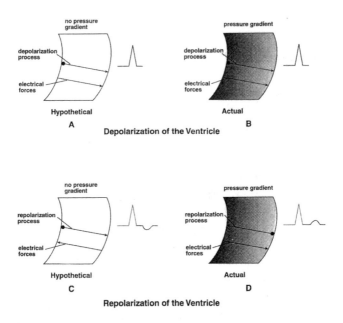

Figure 7-4. The effect of the transmyocardial pressure gradient on the direction of the mean vector representing the QRS complexes and T waves. *A.* In the hypothetical situation, the direction of the depolarization process is directed from endocardium to epicardium. Note there is no transmyocardial pressure gradient (no shading) in this theoretical example. The direction of the depolarization *process* is illustrated by arrow •→. The direction of the *electrical force* that is produced is the same. It is illustrated by arrow →. *B.* The pressure gradient across the ventricular myocardium is illustrated by the shading of the muscle wall. The direction of the depolarization *process* and the *electrical force* it produces is not altered from the direction shown in *A*. *C.* In this hypothetical situation, the direction of the repolarization process is directed from endocardium to epicardium. Note there is no transmyocardial pressure gradient (no shading) in this theoretical example. The direction of the repolarization *process* is illustrated by arrow •→. Note that the direction of the *electrical force* it produces is illustrated by arrow ← and that it is directed in an opposite direction, making an inverted or negative T wave. *D.* The pressure gradient across the ventricular myocardium is illustrated by the shading of the muscle wall. It has been postulated that the repolarization *process* begins in the epicardium because the high pressure in the endocardium delays the repolarization process in that area (2). The *repolarization process* is illustrated by arrow ←•; the direction of the *electrical force* it produces is illustrated by arrow →. This produces an upright or positive T wave.

ventricles when the ventricular pressure is higher than it was when the initial portion of the QRS complex was produced. It seems likely, as suggested by Grant, that the transmyocardial pressure gradient, in which the pressure is higher in the endocardial region than it is in the epicardial region, must play a role in influencing the repolarization process to be directed from the epicardium to the endocardium (2). The higher pressure in the endocardial region seems to delay the repolarization process in that region of the ventricles. The influence of the transmyocardial pressure gradient on the repolarization process is shown in Figure 7-4D.

Note in the discussion of the depolarization of the ventricles, it was possible to attribute a designated portion of the QRS complex to the depolarization of a specific anatomic parts of the ventricles. For example, the initial 0.01 second of the QRS complex was stated to be produced by the depolarization of the left middle portion of the inner surface of the interventricular septum. No such claims can be made for any part of the T wave and the electrical forces that produce the entire T wave, are usually dealt with as a mean force and represented by a mean T vector.

The direction and size of the mean T vector is altered by many conditions, including ischemia, left and right ventricular hypertrophy, pericarditis, and drugs. Also, it must always be remembered that the direction of repolarization is predetermined by the direction of depolarization. This phenomenon must be appreciated especially when there is left or right conduction system block, because in such cases it is necessary to separate primary T wave abnormalities due to disease from secondary T wave "abnormalities" due to the altered sequence of depolarization.

THE S-T SEGMENT

The S-T segment is usually flat and located at the level of the baseline in the normal electrocardiogram. That is to say, it is on the same horizontal line as the T-P segment (see Fig. 7-5A).

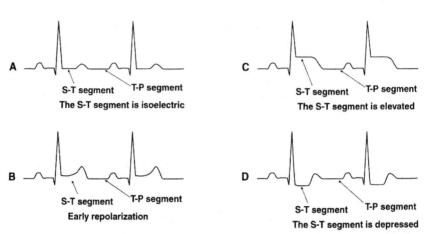

Figure 7-5 The location of the S-T segment. *A.* The usual location of the normal S-T segment. It is on the line with the T-P segment. *B.* The S-T segment may be normally elevated. When it is, the mean spatial S-T segment vector is parallel with the mean T vector. The S-T segment displacement is part of the T wave in that it is the result of the forces of repolarization. Note that the T wave is large in such cases. There are, however, abnormal causes for a mean S-T segment vector that is parallel with the mean T vector. These conditions, including diastolic overload of the left ventricle and subendocardial ischemia, are discussed later in the text. *C.* The S-T segment may be displaced upward and the T wave may not be prominent. As discussed later, the cause is determined more accurately when the spatial characteristics of the forces producing the S-T segment are diagrammed. *D.* The S-T segment may be displaced downward. This is usually abnormal and may be caused by several different conditions. As discussed later, the cause is determined more accurately when the spatial characteristics of the forces producing the S-T segment are diagrammed.

Some normal individuals repolarize their ventricles *earlier* than others and produce electrical forces during the S-T segment (see Fig. 7-5B). A vector representing these forces is directed relatively parallel to the mean T vector. When there is no other evidence of heart disease this finding is referred to as early repolarization. This type of S-T segment displacement may also be abnormal, occurring with diastolic overload of the left ventricle and with endocardial ischemia of the left ventricle. On the other hand, some individuals may repolarize their ventricles *later* than others, producing long Q-T intervals. This finding may be a signal that ventricular arrhythmias, syncope, and sudden death may occur in such patients. This important subject will be discussed later in the book.

The S-T segment may be elevated as shown in Figure 7-2C. This abnormality may be caused by epicardial injury due to myocardial ischemia or pericarditis. The cause of the S-T segment displacement is determined more accurately by identifying the spatial direction of the electrical forces that produces the abnormality. This will be discussed in detail in subsequent chapters.

The S-T segment may be displaced downward (see Figure 7-5D). This is usually abnormal. There are many causes of this abnormality, and the etiology is determined more accurately by diagramming the spatial direction of the forces that produce it. This will be discussed in detail in subsequent chapters.

U WAVES

The normal U wave is produced by the repolarization of the His-Purkinje system. The spatial direction of the small normal U wave cannot be determined from the 12-lead routine tracing because it is usually not seen in all 12 leads. Antzelevitch and his associates believe that abnormally large U waves are the result of split or interrupted T waves (3). Accordingly, they are caused by an abnormal repolarization process in the ventricles. These abnormal U waves will be discussed in Chapter 21.

Abnormally large U waves, or inverted U waves, almost always indicate disease such as hypertension, coronary disease, valve disease, cardiomyopathy, or hypo-kalemia.

OTHER IMPORTANT WAVES

There are four additional waves that must be specifically looked for. Although they are seldom seen, they must not be overlooked or misinterpreted, because they are diagnostic of serious conditions.

Delta waves signify preexcitation of the ventricles (Fig. 2-2) (4). This abnormality is responsible for episodes of supraventricular tachycardia and atrial fibrillation (see Chapter 23).

Osborn waves are due to post-excitation of the ventricles (Figure 2-2) (4). This abnormality is usually caused by hypothermia (see Chapter 23).

Epsilon waves are little wiggles in the S-T segments of leads V_1–V_3 (4). They occur in patients with arrhythmogenic right ventricular dysplasia and other right ventricular abnormalities such as right ventricular infarction (Fig. 2-2). This abnormality may cause treacherous arrhythmias. These waves are discussed in Chapter 23.

Brugada waves are peculiar S-T segment abnormalities in lead V_1-V_3 and are called noncoronary S-T segment displacement (4) (Fig. 2-2). They are often associated with right conduction system abnormalities. They may be responsible for ventricular arrhythmias and sudden death. These waves are discussed in Chapter 23.

REFERENCES

1. Durrer E. Electrical aspects of human cardiac activity: a clinical physiological approach to excitation and stimulation. Cardiovasc Res 1968;2:1.

2. Grant RP. *Clinical Electrocardiography: The spatial vector approach*. New York: The Blakiston Division, McGraw-Hill Book Co Inc, 1957:69.

3. Antzelevitch C. The M cell. J Cardiovasc Pharmacol Ther 1997; 2:73–76.

4. Hurst JW. Naming of the waves in the ECG, with a brief account of their genesis. Circulation 1998;98:1937–1942.

Chapter 8

Memory No. 6: Leads Used to Measure the Direction and Size of the Electrical Forces Generated by the Heart

Lord Kelvin, who was quoted in the preface, is quoted again here for emphasis. His statement, uttered in the last part of the 19th century, is used here to encourage the reader to examine the measuring system used in electrocardiography.

> When you can measure what you are speaking about, and express it in numbers, you know something about it; but when you cannot measure it, when you cannot express it in numbers, your knowledge is of a meager and unsatisfactory kind: it may be the beginning of knowledge, but you have scarcely, in your thoughts, advanced to the stage of *science* (1).

Over the years, different devices have been used to record and measure the electrical forces of the heart. Waller used a mercury capillary electrometer and Einthoven used an improved galvanometer (see Chapter 2). Today we use a direct writing electronic machine. The record the modern machine produces is not as accurate as the record made with the old string galvanometer, but the modern machine does produce a tracing that is instantly available and is sufficiently accurate for clinical purposes.

The connection of the individual to the machine was not always as easy as it is today. Waller and Einthoven had their subjects place each of their arms and one foot in separate buckets of saline. They attached one end of a wire to each of the buckets and the other ends of the wires to the electrocardiograph machine. Today one simply attaches electrodes to the patient's skin. Wires are then used to connect the electrodes to the machine. The location of the electrodes on the body and their connections to the machine create *leads*. The word lead has many meanings. The word used here, as defined in the dictionary, means *an electrical conductor (usually a wire) conveying current from a source to a place of use* (2). The leads are specifically defined and are used to measure the spatial direction and size of the electrical forces that produce the deflections that compose the electrocardiogram.

The use of leads to record the electrical forces produced by the heart is like photographing a person's head from a number of different vantage points. If the camera is placed far enough away from the person, there will be no distortion of the images seen on the film. The images on the film will be different because the camera "views" the person's head from different positions. On the other hand, the image on the film will be distorted if the camera is placed too close to the person being photographed. For example, the photograph of the person's chin might be abnormally large because of the nearness of the camera.

LEADS USED IN CLINICAL ELECTROCARDIOGRAPHY

Einthoven's Bipolar Extremity Leads

The location of the electrodes on the body must be memorized because they were originally arranged arbitrarily and named by Einthoven.

Lead I: The electrode that is placed on the right arm is attached by a wire that is connected to the negative pole of the electrocardiograph machine and the electrode that is placed on the left arm is attached to a wire that is connected to the positive pole of the machine. The machine records the *difference* in electrical potential that is recorded at the two sites. This lead is illustrated in Figure 8-1A.

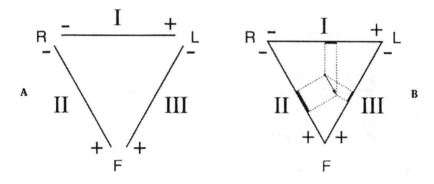

Figure 8-1 *A*. Einthoven's bipolar extremity leads. R = right arm. L = left arm. F = (foot) leg. The positive (+) and negative (−) signs imply that a wire is connected from the extremity to the positive (+) or negative (−) pole of the electrocardiograph machine. *B*. Einthoven's equilateral triangle. Note that the electrode on each extremity is electrically equidistant from the center of the triangle, which is considered to be where the electricity originates. The electrical force in this example is parallel to lead axis II. Note how it projects onto lead axes I, II and III. (*Source*: Hurst JW. *Cardiovascular Diagnosis: The Initial Examination*. St. Louis: Mosby-Year Book, Inc, 1993:204. The author, J.W.H., owns the copyright.)

Lead II: The electrode that is placed on the right arm is attached by a wire that is connected to the negative pole of the electrocardiograph machine, and the electrode that is placed on a leg is attached to a wire that is connected to the positive pole of the machine. The machine records the *difference* in the electrical potential that is recorded at the two sites. This lead is illustrated in Figure 8-1A.

Lead III: The electrode that is placed on the left arm is attached by a wire that is connected to the negative pole of the electrocardiograph machine, and the electrode placed on a leg is attached to a wire that is connected to the positive pole of the machine. The machine records the difference in the electrical potential that is recorded at the two sites. This lead is illustrated in Figure 8-1A.

The imaginary lines connecting the two electrodes that compose each of the leads are called *lead axes*. The word axis also has many meanings. The word, as it is used here, simply indicates a line that connects two points.

Einthoven's equilateral triangle and Einthoven's law

Einthoven was an excellent mathematician and envisioned the *equilateral* triangle (See fig. 8-1B). The three sides of the triangle are composed of the imaginary lead axes created by leads I, II, and III. Obviously, the equilateral triangle does not relate to anatomic structures because if anatomy is considered, the axes of leads II and III would be longer than the axis of lead I and the triangle would not be equilateral. The equilateral triangle is not related to anatomy; it is an *electrical equilateral triangle*. Einthoven placed the origin of electrical forces of the heart in the center of the triangle (see Fig. 8-1B) and recognized that *electrically speaking* the electrode on the right and left arms are no closer to the origin of electrical force than is the electrode on the leg. This is true because the magnitude of electrical potential is determined by the formula shown in Figure 8-2.

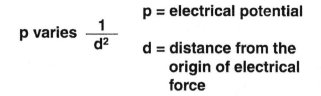

$$\text{p varies } \frac{1}{d^2}$$

p = electrical potential

d = distance from the origin of electrical force

Figure 8-2 Electrical potential varies inversely with the square of the distance the measuring device is from the source of electricity. This is the mathematical proof that the arms and legs are electrically equidistant from the source of electricity that they record. (*Source*: Burch VG, Winsor EA. *A Primer of Electrocardiography*. Philadelphia: Lea & Febiger, 1945:21. Public domain.)

Einthoven's law states that the electrocardiographic deflection seen in lead I, plus the electrocardiographic deflection seen in lead III, equals the electrocardiographic deflection seen in lead II.* This law is based on the work of Kirchoff, which states that "the algebraic sum of all electrical forces flowing to a single point in a network is equal to zero" (3). Einthoven's law is useful when an artifact distorts the recording and prevents the interpretation of the P, QRS, and T waves in one of the bipolar leads; the poorly recorded deflections can be constructed mathematically if the deflections on two leads can be identified.

Einthoven's equilateral triangle is commonly used as a graphic display system. Figure 8–1B illustrates the projection of a single electrical force onto lead axes I, II, and III. The heart, of course, creates an infinite number of electrical forces but it is wise to begin with the study of a single force.

When an electrical force is directed toward an electrode that is attached to the positive pole of the recording machine

---

* Einthoven originally arranged the bipolar extremity leads so that the deflection on lead I plus the deflections on leads II plus the deflection on III equaled zero. He later reversed the polarity of lead axis II so that with the new arrangement, a deflection on lead I plus the deflection on lead III equals the deflection in lead II.

it, produces an upright deflection; and when it is directed toward an electrode that is attached to the negative pole of the recording machine, it produces a downward deflection. When an electrical force is directed midway between the two electrodes of a bipolar lead axis, it will produce zero deflection.

Bayley's Triaxial System (A Modification of Einthoven's Triangle)

Robert Bayley graduated from Emory University School of Medicine. His house staff training was at the University Hospital in Ann Arbor, Michigan. During his four years at Ann Arbor he became closely associated with Dr. Frank Wilson. He studied with Wilson and contributed significantly to our knowledge of electrocardiography. In order to make a more usable display system, he moved the lead axes comprising Einthoven's triangle so they would pass through the origin of electrical activity (see Fig. 8-3A). While doing so, he carefully

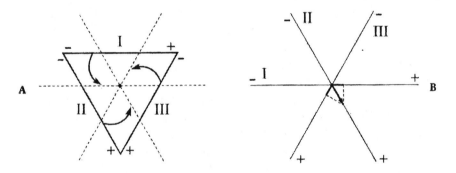

Figure 8-3 Bayley's triaxial system. *A*. The lead axes created by Einthoven are transposed so that they pass through the center of electrical activity of the heart. The inclination of the lead axes are maintained. *B*. Note in this figure that the projections of the electrical forces on lead I, II, III that were displayed in Figure 8–1B remain the same in this figure. (Source: Hurst JW. *Cardiovascular Diagnosis: The Initial Examination*. St. Louis: Mosby-Year Book, Inc, 1993: 206. The author, J.W.H., owns the copyright.)

maintained the same spatial orientation of the lead axes. Note how the electrical force illustrated in Figure 8-3B projects the same amount on each of the leads as it projected on the same leads in Figure 8-1B.

Wilson's Unipolar Leads

Each of the bipolar extremity leads measures the difference between the electrical potential that influences each of the two electrodes that compose the leads. During the 1940's the search was on to develop a unipolar lead so that the electrical potential could be recorded at one electrode site. Wilson created the unipolar lead system by using Einthoven's law, which was based on Kircoff's law. Wilson placed an electrode on each arm and a leg and pulled the wires together and called the union the *central terminal*. He attached the central terminal to the negative pole of the electrocardiograph machine and, using another wire, attached the *exploring electrode* to the positive pole of the electrocardiograph machine (see Fig. 8-4). The central terminal, following Einthoven's law, is almost neutral at all times so the exploring electrode is influenced solely by the electrical potential located at that body site. The exploring electrode could then be placed on the extremities or on the chest surface.

Wilson's Unipolar Chest Leads

Einthoven used no chest leads. Perhaps this was because his "electrodes" were buckets of saline, which prohibited their use on the chest. When simple electrodes were developed, investigators began to record the electrocardiogram by placing the electrodes on the anterior chest wall. Initially, they connected an arm electrode to the negative pole of the electrocardiograph machine and connected the chest electrode, which was placed at *one* spot on the chest surface, to the positive pole of the electrocardiograph machine. The investigators eventually created the six precordial chest leads. As the investigators searched for the best leads, they used CR, CL, and CF leads.

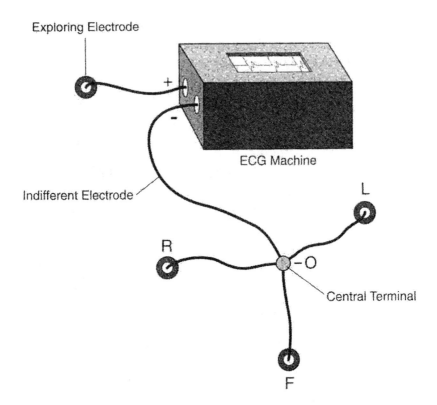

Exploring Electrode

ECG Machine

Indifferent Electrode

L

R

O

Central Terminal

F

Figure 8-4 Wilson's unipolar lead arrangement. R = right arm; L = left arm; F = foot (leg). (Source: Hurst JW. *Cardiovascular Diagnosis: The Initial Examination*. St. Louis: Mosby-Year Book, Inc, 1993:207. The author, J.W.H., owns the copyright.)

They were all bipolar leads; the C referred to the chest, and R, L, and F identified the extremity that was used to create the bipolar chest lead. After much research the Wilson unipolar chest lead was proved to be superior to bipolar chest leads. It is called a V lead because V is the symbol for potential. The locations of the six chest electrode positions are shown in Figure 8-5. The electrode for lead V_1 is located in the fourth intercostal space adjacent to the right side of the sternum. The elec-

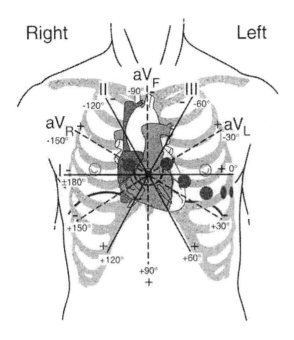

Figure 8-5 The location of the chest electrodes (see text). Source: Hurst JW. *Cardiovascular Diagnosis: The Initial Examination*. St. Louis: Mosby-Year Book, Inc, 1993:210. The author, J.W.H., owns the copyright.)

trode lead V_2 is located in the fourth intercostal space adjacent to the left side of the sternum. The electrode for lead V_3 is located at the midpoint of an imaginary line connecting the electrode for leads V_2 and V_4. The electrode for lead V_4 is located in the fifth intercostal space on the midclavicular line. The electrode for lead V_5 is located on the anterior axillary line at the same level as the electrode for lead V_4. The electrode for lead V_6 is located on the midaxillary line at the same level as the electrodes for leads V_4 and V_5. The imaginary lead axes for the chest leads can be visualized by drawing a line from the chest electrode through the site of the origin of the electrical force to the other side of the chest.

The Unipolar Extremity Leads

Wilson's unipolar extremity leads were used during the early 1940s. It was necessary to amplify the electrical signals from the extremities by about one third in order for the potential to register the same amount on the unipolar extremity leads as they registered on the bipolar leads. This was desirable because Wilson wanted to establish a mathematical relationship between the bipolar extremity leads and the unipolar extremity leads. The unipolar extremity leads were called VR, VL, and VF. Such amplification was not needed when the Wilson unipolar lead was used to record the chest leads, because the electrodes were near the heart and large complexes were recorded.

Legend holds that amplifers "went to war" (World War II) and the Wilson unipolar extremity leads could not be used because the electrical potential could not be amplified. Emanual Goldberger discovered how to augment the electrical units of the Wilson unipolar leads without using an amplifier. He simply broke the connection from the extremity to the central terminal when the exploring electrode was placed on that extremity (see Fig. 8-6).

The Goldberger augmented extremity leads are labeled aV_R, aV_L, and aV_F; the letter a is the symbol for augmented. The axes of the augmented extremity leads bisect the angles produced by the bipolar leads displayed in Bayley's triaxial system and produce the hexaxial reference system (see Fig. 8-7).

The deflections recorded from the extremities using Goldberger's unipolar augmented leads are not identical to the deflections that are recorded using Wilson unipolar extremity leads. The differences, however, are not of clinical significance. What is fortunate is that the deflections that are recorded using Goldberger leads are augmented about the right amount so that a mathematical relationship can be established between deflections recorded using the augmented unipolar extremity leads and the deflections using Einthoven bipolar leads.

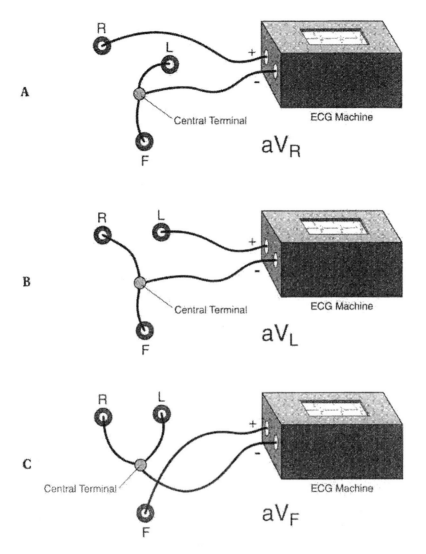

Figure 8-6 Goldberger's unipolar extremity lead arrangement (see text). R = right arm; L = left arm; F = foot (leg). (*Source*: Hurst JW. *Cardiovascular Diagnosis: The Initial Examination*. St. Louis: Mosby-Year Book, Inc, 1993:208. The author, J.W.H., owns the copyright.)

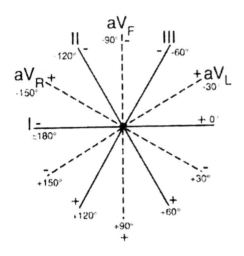

Figure 8-7 The hexaxial reference system. This figure illustrates how Goldberger's augmented extremity lead system relates to the triaxial system of Bayley. The angles between axes are 30°, and for every bipolar lead axis there is an unipolar lead axis that is perpendicular to it. This fact will be used later when the method of determining the direction of electrical forces is discussed. Note the number of degrees listed at the end of the lead axes; these numbers are used to designate the frontal plane direction of electrical forces. (*Source*: Hurst JW. *Cardiovascular Diagnosis: The Initial Examination*. St. Louis: Mosby-Year Book, Inc 1993:209. The author, J.W.H., owns the copyright.)

Special Leads

Special leads are used for special purposes.

Fontaine leads are used to identify epsilon waves (4). The right arm electrode is placed on the upper part of the sternum and, the left arm lead is placed on the end of the sternum, and the leg electrode is placed at the cardiac apex. The sensitivity of the electrocardiograph machine is doubled, and the recording is made using leads I, II, and III. This system of recording is used when the clinician suspects arrhythmogenic right ventricular dysplasia and is prospecting for epsilon waves (4).

Some individuals use *leads* V_3R and V_4R in the search for S-T segment elevation that accompanies right ventricular infarction. These chest electrodes are placed on the right side of the chest using the same guidelines that were used when electrodes are placed on the left side of the chest. *These leads are not needed when one understands the use of vector concepts discussed in this book (5).* Also, an error can be made by concluding that elevated S-T segments recorded in V_3R and V_4R always indicate right ventricular infarction, because septal infarcts and subendocardial injury can create the same abnormality.

An *esophageal lead* is sometimes used in the search for P waves in patients with arrhythmias. While such a lead is valuable, it is not used as much today as it was used formerly.

THE RECORDING ITSELF

The leads described above produce the conduit by which the electricity produced by the heart is transmitted to the electrocardiograph machine. The modern direct-writer records the deflections on a strip of moving paper. The paper speed is 25

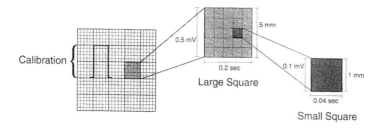

Figure 8-8 Paper used in modern electrocardiograph machine. Note that the machine is calibrated so that the stylus of the machine will rise two large squares (10 millimeters). The paper speed is 25 millimeters per second. (*Source*: Hurst JW. *Cardiovascular Diagnosis: The Initial Examination*. St. Louis: Mosby-Year Book, Inc, 1993: 203. The author, J.W.H., owns the copyright.)

millimeters per second. The grid that is imprinted on the paper has the characteristics shown in Figure 8-8.

As will be discussed in Chapter 10, the lead axes are used to measure the direction and magnitude of the electrical forces that create the deflections seen in the recording. It is far more scientific to identify and measure the direction and size of the electrical forces that produce the deflections than it is to memorize the shapes of the deflections.

REFERENCES

1. William Thomson, Lord Kelvin. Popular Lectures and Addresses, 1891–1894.

2. Oxford American Dictionary. New York: Avon Books, 1980:376.

3. Burch G, Winsor T. A Primer of Electrocardiography. Philadelphia: Lea & Febiger, 1945:53.

4. Hurst JW. Naming of the waves in the ECG, with a brief account of their genesis. Circulation 1998;98:1937–1942.

5. Hurst JW. Detection of right ventricular myocardial infarction associated with inferior myocardial infarction from the standard 12-lead electrocardiogram. Heart Disease and Stroke 1993;2: 464–467.

Chapter 9

The Fusion of Six Memories

It is necessary to fuse the six memories discussed on the previous pages of this book *into one image with six parts*. The memories include the use of vectors; the electrical activity of an isolated myocyte; the attributes of a volume conductor; the anatomy of the heart, including the heart chambers, coronary arteries, and the conduction system; depolarization and repolarization of the atria and ventricles, the S-T segment, U waves; and the leads used to measure the direction and size of electrical forces. These overlapping images must be superimposed one on the other and *used as part of the thought process* associated with the interpretation of every electrocardiogram (see Fig. 9-1) (1). Furthermore, this cognitive action must be practiced and practiced until a state of fluency is achieved.

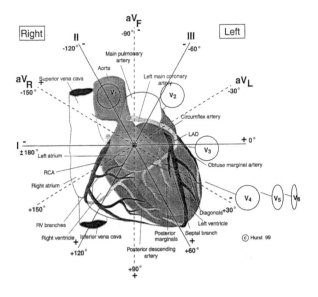

Figure 9-1 The superimposition of memories needed to interpret electrocardiograms. This figure illustrates the location of the chambers of the heart, the coronary arteries, and the lead axes that are used to determine the size and direction of the electrical forces that produce the electrocardiogram. Not shown are the characteristics of a vector, the electrical activity of a single myocyte, information about the chest as a volume conductor; the anatomy of the conduction system; the depolarization and repolarization of the atria and ventricles, and the S-T and U waves. The reader should, however, include these important images in the thought process used to interpret electrocardiograms. Obviously, this single diagram does not indicate the location of the heart and its component parts of all individuals. This is true because the atria and ventricles may be located more vertically in some individuals and more horizontally in others. The location of the coronary arteries is even more variable. Accordingly, a single diagram can only teach the *concept* that should be used in the thought process needed to interpret electrocardiograms. RCA = right coronary artery; LAD = left anterior descending coronary artery.

(*Source*: The basic illustration appeared in Hurst JW. Methods used to interpret the 12-lead electrocardiogram: Pattern memorization versus the use of vector concepts. Clin Cardiol 2000;23:4–13. Used with permission. The sites for the location of the precordial electrodes have been added.)

REFERENCE

1.   Hurst JW. Methods used to interpret the 12-lead electrocardio-
     gram: Pattern memorization versus the use of vector concepts.
     Clin Cardiol 2000;23:4–13.

Chapter 10

How to Measure the Electrical Forces Created by the Heart

The spatial direction and amplitude of the electrical forces that create the deflections seen in the electrocardiogram must be determined. These measurements are accomplished by studying the electrocardiographic deflections recorded in the 12-lead electrocardiogram.

GRANT'S METHOD OF MEASURING THE DIRECTION OF ELECTRICAL FORCES

The spatial direction of the electrical forces produced by the heart can be determined by using the two steps described below (1).

Step 1. This step is used to determine the frontal plane projection of the electrical forces. *When an electrical force, represented as a vector, is directed parallel to a given extremity lead axis, it records its largest deflection in that axis. When an electrical force is directed perpendicular to a given extremity lead axis, it will record its smallest deflection on that axis.* In making this calculation, the largest and smallest deflections are determined by estimating the *area* subtended by the complex being studied.

The precise number of degrees an electrical force, which is represented by a vector, is deviated to the right or left or up and down can be determined by matching the direction of the electrical force to the degrees indicated on the hexaxial display system (see Fig. 10-1). Note the numbers inscribed at the end of each extremity lead axis. The number inscribed at the right end of lead axis I is zero. The numbers located at the end of the extremity lead axes in the upper half of the display system are $-30°$, $-60°$, $-90°$, $-120°$, $-150°$, and $\pm180°$. The numbers located at the end of the extremity lead axes in the lower half of the display system are $+30°$, $+60°$, $+90°$, $+120°$, $+150°$, and $\pm180°$.

The calculation of the frontal plane directions of an electrical force by the method described above is fairly accurate; with practice the intraobserver and interobserver variance will be about $5°$.

An example demonstrating the use of step 1 is shown in Figure 10-1. The largest deflection is noted in lead I and the smallest deflection is seen in lead aV_F. Accordingly, the vector is directed at $0°$.

Step 2. This step is used to determine the anterior or posterior direction of electrical forces. *This step must not be taken without first determining the frontal plane direction of an electrical force* (see step 1 above). The largest precordial lead deflection, as determined by area, *cannot* be used to indicate that an electrical force is parallel to that particular precordial lead axis. This is because the electrical potential varies inversely with the square of the distance between the origin of the force

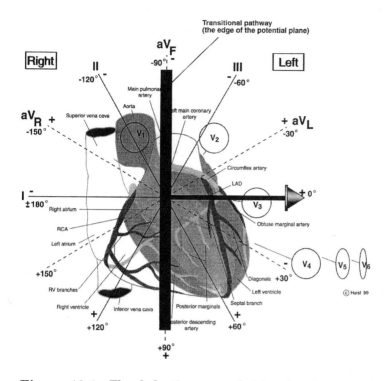

Figure 10-1   The deflections recorded by the six extremity leads are used to determine the frontal plane direction of electrical forces. Suppose the area subtended by the deflection being studied is upright and largest in lead I and smallest in lead aV_F. The vector representing the electrical force would be directed at zero degrees to the left because it would be parallel with lead axis I, perpendicular to lead axis aV_F, and directed toward the positive pole of lead I. As shown in the diagram, the number of degrees an electrical force can be directed in the frontal plane is shown at the end of the bipolar and unipolar extremity lead axes. Note the location of the transitional pathway.

(*Source*: The body of this illustration appeared in Hurst JW. Methods used to interpret the 12-lead electrocrdiogram: Pattern memorization versus the use of vector concepts. Clin Cardiol 2000;23:4–13. Used with permission.)

and the location where the measurement is made. Therefore, the chest electrodes are more influenced by a unit of electrical force than the extremity electrodes are influenced by the same unit. It is possible to use the smallest precordial lead deflection to make the measurement because it is recorded from the transitional pathway. Remember the following important points: the transitional pathway, located on the surface of the chest, represents the edge of the zero potential plane that is perpendicular to the direction of the electrical force (see Chapter 5). Therefore, keeping the frontal plane direction of the electrical force in mind, the vector representing the electrical force is directed anteriorly or posteriorly until the edge of its potential plane, the transitional pathway, passes through one of the precordial electrode positions that reveals the smallest deflection. The smallest deflection is determined by adding algebraically the area above the baseline to area below the baseline. At times, of course, the transition from negative to positive will be located between two of the precordial electrode positions.

Suppose, for example, after establishing the frontal plane direction of an electrical force, as shown in Figure 10-1, the interpreter notes that the deflections in leads V_1, V_2, and V_3 are resultantly negative and the deflections in leads V_4, V_5, and V_6 are resultantly positive; the transitional pathway can be visualized as being between leads V_3 and V_4. The vector representing the direction of electrical force would be directed about 45° posteriorly (Fig. 10-2).

The determination of the anterior-posterior direction of electrical forces is not as accurate as the determination of the frontal plane directions, and the margin of error is about ±15°. No specific number of degrees can be assigned to the chest lead axes as can be done for the extremity lead axes. The interpreter must simply visualize the chest and the direction of the frontal plane vector and then estimate the location of the zero potential plane and recognize that the vector is perpendicular to that plane. Figure 10-3 has been designed to help the reader develop the spatial sense needed to accomplish the goal.

This approach should be used to determine the direction

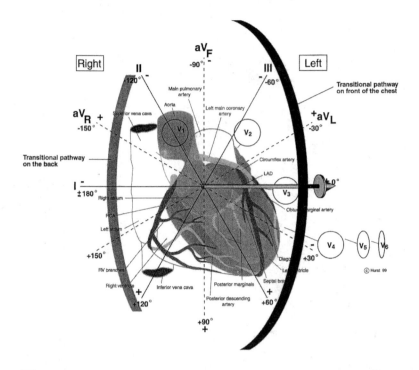

Figure 10-2 The deflections recorded by the six precordial leads are used to determine the anterior or posterior direction of electrical forces. The frontal plane direction of the vector is at 0°. Suppose the complex, or the portion of the complex being studied, is resultantly zero between leads V_3 and V_4. Should that be the case, one could assume that the vector would be directed about 45° posteriorly. Note the location of the transitional pathway.

(*Source*: The body of this illustration appeared in Hurst JW. Methods used to interpret the 12-lead electrocardiogram: Pattern memorization versus the use of vector concepts. Clin Cardiol 2000;23:4–13. Used with permission.)

of the vectors representing the mean P wave, first and last half of the P wave, mean QRS complex, initial 0.01 second of the QRS complex, initial and terminal 0.04 second of the QRS complex, mean S-T segment, and T wave. As will be discussed later, the vectors representing these parts of the complexes

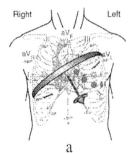
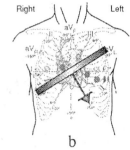
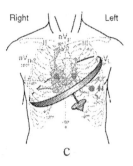

a

b

c

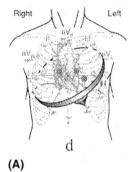
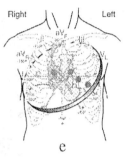
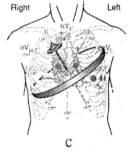

d

e

f

(A)

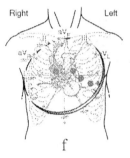

a

b

c

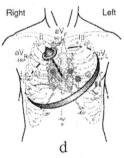
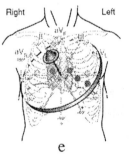
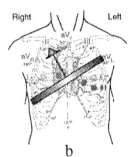
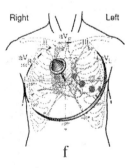

d

e

f

(B)

Figure 10-3 Calculation of the anterior or posterior direction of an electrical force (vector). This diagram is included in an effort to assist the reader visualize how to deduce the number of degrees a vector is directed anteriorly or posteriorly. A. Assume that the frontal plane direction of an electrical force (vector) represented by an arrow is largest and positive in lead axis II. The arrow representing the electrical force (vector) would be directed parallel with lead axis II; it would be directed toward the electrode that is attached to the positive pole of the electrocardiograph machine and away from the electrode that is attached to the negative pole of the electrocardiograph machine. The vector would be directed at $+60°$ in the frontal plane. (a) When the transtional pathway passes through electrode position V_1, the electrical force (vector) reprsented by an arrow is directed about 10° to 20° anteriorly. (b) When the transitional pathway passes through electrode position V_2, the electrical force (vector) represented by an arrow is parallel with the frontal plan. (c) When the transitional pathway passes through electrode position V_3, the electrical force (vector) represented by an arrow is directed about 20° to 30° posteriorly. (d) When the transitional pathway passes through electrode position V_4, the electrical force (vector) represented by an arrow is directed 40° to 50° posteriorly. (e) When the transitional pathway passes through electrode position V_5, the electrical force (vector) represented by an arrow is directed 60° to 70° posteriorly. (f) When the transitional pathway passes through electrode position V_6, the electrical force (vector) represented by an arrow is directed 80° to 90° posteriorly. B. Imagine that the frontal plane direction of the electrical force (vector) is largest but negative in lead axis II. The arrow would be directed parallel to lead axis II; it is directed away from the electrode that is attached to the positive pole of the electrocardiograph machine. The vector would be directed $-120°$ in the frontal plane. (a) When the transitional pathway passes through electrode position V_1, the electrial force (vector) represented by an arrow will be directed 10° to 20° posteriorly. (b) When the transitional pathway passes through electrode position V_2, the electrical force (vector) represented by an arrow will be directed parallel with the frontal plane. (c) When the transitional pathway passes through electrode position V_3, the electrical force (vector) represented by an arrow will be directed about 20° to 30° anteriorly. (d) When the transitional pathway passes through electrode position V_4, the electrical force (vector) represented by an arrow will be directed 40° to 50° anteriorly. (e) When the transitional pathway passes through electrode position V_5, the electrical force (vector) represented by an arrow will be directed 60° to 70° anteriorly. (f) When the transitional pathway passes through electrode position V_6, the electrical force (vector) represented by an arrow will be directed 80° to 90° anteriorly.
(*Source*: Hurst JW. *Cardiovascular Diagnosis: The Initial Examination*. St. Louis: Mosby-Year Book, Inc. 1993:213–214. The author, J.W.H., owns the copyright.)

are called diagnostic cardiac vectors because they become abnormal in response to certain diseases.

SOME HELPFUL SUGGESTIONS

Note that lead axis aV_F is perpendicular to lead axis I, lead
axis aV_L is perpendicular to lead axis II, and lead axis aV_R is
perpendicular to lead axis III. When calculating the frontal
plane direction of an electrical force it is useful to identify the
lead axis in which the smallest deflection is found and to immediately check the lead axis that is perpendicular to that axis
because the largest deflection should be seen in that axis.

The art of interpolating should be perfected. Suppose the
interpreter identifies the smallest deflection in a certain lead.
For example, it might be determined that the smallest deflection is in lead aV_L, but the deflection is just slightly positive.
The interpreter realizes that the electrical force would be isoelectric (zero) in lead aV_L if the vector were directed at exactly
$+60°$. Because the smallest deflection is just barely positive
in lead aV_L the interpreter should assume the vector is directed at $+55°$ rather than $+60°$.

The following discussion is included here so the reader
can review these points:

> The zero potential plane is perpendicular to the direction
> of the electrical force that is represented by a vector.
> The zero potential plane intersects the surface of the
> body where, on the surface of the chest, it becomes
> the transitional pathway. The reader should use a
> piece of cardboard to represent the zero potential
> plane. The reader should then pierce the center of
> the cardboard with a pencil; the pencil represents an
> electrical force. Note that the cardboard is perpen-
> dicular to the direction of the pencil.
> Assume the hole in the cardboard is the origin of the elec-
> trical force and pretend that the origin of the electri-
> cal force is located in the center of the heart.

Establish an arbitrary frontal plane direction for the pencil. For example, suppose the pencil is directed at zero and is parallel with the frontal plane.

Suppose the smallest resultant precordial deflection of the QRS complex is located between lead V_3 and V_4. Now rotate the cardboard until the edge of the cardboard passes between electrodes V_3 and V_4 where the resultantly smallest deflection is seen. Now note the direction of the pencil and estimate the number of degrees the vector is rotated posteriorly.

To emphasize what was stated earlier: there is no mathematical relationship between the six precordial leads as there is between the extremity leads because the precordial leads are too near the heart. There is no Einthoven law for the chest leads. Therefore, the interpreter must learn to visualize the chest and estimate the number of degrees the electrical forces are directed from the frontal plane (see Fig. 10-3). This limitation is compounded when one realizes that the electrode placement on the chest varies considerably depending on the size of the thorax. Because of these limitations, the margin of error in determining the anterior and posterior direction of an electrical force is ±15°.

MEASURING THE AMPLITUDE OF AN ELECTRICAL FORCE

The method of measuring the amplitude of the deflections will be discussed in the chapters dealing with normal and abnormal electrocardiograms. Here it should be emphasized that the *direction* of an electrical force is computed by using the size of the *area* subtended by the part of the deflection being studied and that the measurement of the *amplitude* of a deflection is accomplished by measuring the *length* of the deflection above or below the baseline of the electrocardiogram.

When the direction of the mean vector representing the

QRS complexes and direction of the mean vector representing the T waves are calculated, the observer should use the area subtended by the complexes to make the calculation. When doing so, the length of the arrows should reflect the relative size of the two measurements. That is, if the area under the QRS is twice as large as it is under the T wave, the mean QRS vector should be drawn to be twice as long as the mean T vector. The amplitude of the QRS complex is a different measurement entirely and is determined by the thickness of the ventricular wall as well as body build. This measurement is made by measuring the height or depth of the QRS complexes. The normal amplitude of the QRS complex is discussed in Chapter 12.

MEASURING THE DURATION OF THE WAVES

Measuring the duration of the P wave, P-R interval, QRS complex, and the Q-T interval are all part of measuring and are discussed in Chapter 12.

COMMUNICATING THE CHARACTERISTICS OF THE DEFLECTIONS

Once the method of measuring and diagramming the direction and amplitude of electrical forces has been mastered, it is possible to communicate in a different manner (2). For example, rather than stating that the T wave is low in lead I, inverted in lead aV_R and aV_L, and upright in leads II, III, and aV_F, inverted in lead V_1 and V_2, and upright in leads V_3-V_6, it is possible to state that the mean T vector is directed about $+85°$ in the frontal plane about $10°$ posteriorly. Better still, one can simply draw the mean T vector on the display diagram and say or write nothing else.

Extending the thought, the electrocardiogram should be interpreted in terms of the direction and amplitude of the diagnostic cardiac vectors and the relationship of the vectors to each other.

The words *diagnostic cardiac vectors* are used because these vectors are useful in making cardiac diagnoses. To repeat, the diagnostic cardiac vectors include the mean P vector, vectors representing the first half and second half of the P waves; the mean QRS vector, vectors representing the first 0.01 second of the QRS complexes, the initial 0.04 second of the QRS complexes, and the last .04 second of the QRS complexes; a mean vector representing the S-T segments; and a mean vector representing the T waves. These diagnostic cardiac vectors were so designated after studying vectorcardiograms in which all of the instantaneous electrical forces are recorded. The diagnostic cardiac vectors were chosen because they represent the parts of the vectorcardiograms that are useful in making cardiac diagnoses.

REFERENCES

1.   Grant RP. Spatial vector electrocardiography: A method for calculating the spatial electrical vectors of the heart from conventional leads. Circulation 1950;2:676–695.

2.   Hurst JW. Methods used to interpret the 12-lead electrocardiogram: Pattern memorization versus the use of vector concepts. Clin Cardiol 2000;23:4–13.

Part IV

The Clinician's Use of the Electrocardiogram as a Diagnostic Tool

Chapter 11

The Clinical Use of Electrocardiography

The heart is a versatile organ. It moves, makes noises, creates electricity, and produces symptoms when it is diseased or functions abnormally. All of these attributes are examined routinely when the clinician analyzes the patient's symptoms, interprets the results of a meticulous physical examination, and interprets the electrocardiogram and chest x-ray film (1).

The electrocardiogram is used almost routinely in adult patients and in children when indicated by other clinical information. The clinician must know when the abnormalities found in the electrocardiogram fit the data collected from the history, physical examination, and chest x-ray film. The unskilled physician may believe the abnormalities found in the electrocardiogram fit the other clinical data, whereas a skilled physician may recognize that they do not. When that occurs, the thinking clinician realizes that one of three things has occurred: the data collection process was faulty, the interpretation of the data was not correct, or the patient has two types of heart disease.

The clinician must also know the limitation of the technique. For example, the clinician must know the types of heart disease that can be present when the electrocardiogram is normal. On the other hand, it is important to know the types of heart disease that a normal electrocardiogram unequivocally excludes. Above all, the clinician must know the meaning of the abnormalities seen in a tracing, because some abnormalities have little clinical significance, whereas others are signs of serious disease.

The clinician must always create a differential cardiac diagnosis for each electrocardiogram, even when the tracing is normal. The thoughtful clinician correlates the data collected from other sources with the possible diagnoses suggested by the electrocardiogram. When this is done, the clinician's diagnostic success rate will gradually increase. With continued practice, the clinician should be able to view the electrocardiogram and create a list of diagnostic possibilities that includes the correct cardiac diagnosis most of the time. When the clinician simply describes the characteristic of the deflections, and does not create a differential diagnosis, he or she is not using the procedure as a diagnostic tool. When this is done, as stated in Chapter 1, the clinician is assuming that collection of information alone is thinking, whereas thinking is much more complex than data collection. Thinking, remember, is the rearrangement of information into a new perception. To simply conclude that a wave in the electrocardiogram is upright or inverted is to hang up in the information stage of the thinking–learning process.

THE STEPS USED TO INTERPRET ELECTROCARDIOGRAMS (2)

1. Determine the heart rate and rhythm. When the heart rate and rhythm are abnormal, the interpreter

should not only identify the abnormal rhythm but should create a differential diagnosis that includes the possible causes for the abnormality.

2. Determine the duration of the P-R or P-Q interval, the duration of the QRS complexes, and the Q-T interval. When the measurements are abnormal, the clinician must determine the cause.

3. Diagram the diagnostic cardiac vectors. This includes diagramming the mean P vector, the vectors representing the first and second half of the P wave; the mean QRS vector, vectors representing the first 0.01 second, the first 0.03–0.04 second, and the last 0.03–0.04 second of the QRS complexes; and a mean vector representing the S-T segments and T waves.

Obviously, the interpreter must know the normal direction and amplitude for the diagnostic cardiac vectors as well as the normal relationship of each of the diagnostic cardiac vectors to the other diagnostic cardiac vectors. When the diagnostic cardiac vectors are abnormal, the clinician should be stimulated to determine the cause (see next step).

4. Establish an electrical-anatomic cardiac differential diagnosis. At times the interpreter will indicate that the patient has, for example, left conduction system block or left ventricular hypertrophy. This is proper, but it is only the beginning of the thought process and not the end (see next step).

5. Establish a differential diagnosis of cardiac diseases that could explain the electrical-anatomic diagnosis created in step 4. This moves the thought process a step further. For example, left ventricular hypertrophy due to systolic pressure overload may be caused by aortic valve stenosis of any cause, systemic hypertension due to any cause, and primary hypertrophy of the left ventricle. Left ventricular hypertrophy due to diastolic overload of the left ventricle may be caused by aortic regurgitation or mitral regurgitation of any cause, or it may develop in athletes.

6. Correlate the information identified in the electrocardiogram with other clinical data. This step is extremely important. The clinician must be sufficiently skilled to determine if the electrocardiographic abnormalities are caused
by the condition suggested from analyzing the data collected by other means. A computer readout never does
that, so computers cannot learn or teach; they continue
to make errors over and over again because they cannot
correlate the electrocardiographic abnormalities with the
other clinical data.

The recording of an electrocardiogram is one of the most
commonly performed technical procedures in the practice of
medicine. It is a superb diagnostic tool, but a faulty interpretation may be dangerous and can lead to much suffering. For
example, myocardial infarction may not be recognized because
of an error in the interpretation of the electrocardiogram. Or
an infarction may be diagnosed from the electrocardiogram
when the abnormalities have a more benign cause.

REFERENCES

1. Hurst JW, Branch WT Jr. Physical examination of the heart,
   arteries, and jugular veins. In: Branch WT Jr, Alexander RW,
   Schlant RC, Hurst JW (eds). *Cardiology in Primary Care*. New
   York: McGraw-Hill, 2000:65–91.

2. Hurst JW. *Cardiovascular Diagnosis: The Initial Examination*.
   St. Louis: Mosby, 1993:238–239.

Part V

Surveying the Waves

The Normal Electrocardiogram

Chapter 12

Normal Measurements
With Brief Comments About Abnormal
Measurements

The purpose of this chapter is to describe the range of normal
for the electrocardiographic deflections seen in neonates, ado-
lescents, and adults. Within this context, abnormalities will
become obvious. Accordingly, certain common abnormalities
will be listed, although the details of the abnormalities will be
discussed in later chapters. At the outset it should be emphasized that electrocardiographic abnormalities that lie outside
the normal range are not necessarily important or of clinical
significance; a separate judgment must be made about the abnormalities to conclude that they are important to the patient.

There is a normal range for most biologic phenomena,
and the deflections seen in the electrocardiogram are no exception to that rule. The probability that a measurement is nor-

mal is 100 percent when the measurement falls in the middle
of the distribution curve. It must be remembered, however,
that the probability that a measurement is normal decreases
while the possibility of an abnormality increases when the
measurement falls at the edges of the distribution curve.

WHAT SHOULD BE SEEN AND MEASURED?

Heart Rate and Rhythm

A normal P wave should precede each QRS complex and the
intervals between the QRS complexes should be equally
spaced. When the duration of the R-R interval varies slightly
with inspiration and expiration, the rhythm is called *sinus
arrhythmia.*

The rate can be determined easily by dividing the number
of large squares noted on the electrocardiographic paper that
are contained between two QRS complexes into 300. The normal heart rate in adults is 60 to 90 QRS complexes per minute.
A P wave precedes each QRS complex. When there are fewer
than 60 complexes per minute in the adult, the rate is labeled
sinus bradycardia, and when there are more than 90 complexes per minute in the adult, the rate is labeled *sinus tachycardia.* The heart rate is normally faster in neonates and children than it is in adults.

P waves and QRS complexes should not be called beats or
contractions because, as emphasized repeatedly, the electrical
forces that create the P waves and QRS complexes may or may
not stimulate mechanical contraction of the atria and ventricles. Electrical-mechanical dissociation may occur in the atria
or ventricles. For example, the return of P waves in the tracing
following the reversion of atrial fibrillation to normal does not
guarantee that the atria are contracting. Likewise, electrical-
mechanical dissociation of the ventricles is one of the mechanisms that causes sudden death. In such cases, QRS complexes can be seen in the tracing but the ventricles do not contract.

The interpretation of arrhythmias is not discussed in this book because the method used to decipher rhythm distur- bances is different from the method used to decipher abnor- malities of the P, QRS, S-T, and T waves.

Duration of the Intervals

The duration of the P-R interval is determined by measuring the time interval from the beginning of the P wave to the be- ginning of the QRS complex. The P-Q interval is preferred when it is available to measure. The measurement indicates the amount of time required for the electrical impulse to travel from the sinus node, through the atrial muscle, through the A- V node where it is delayed, down the left and right ventricular conduction systems, to the ventricular myocytes. The normal P-R interval varies with the heart rate: the faster the heart rate, the shorter the P-R interval (see Table 12–1).

The P-R interval is considered to be short when it is 0.12 second or less in the adult, and it is considered to be long when it is greater than 0.20 second. Short P-R intervals may be due to preexcitation of the ventricles (see discussion in Chapter 23) and a P-R interval greater than 0.20 second is considered to be first-degree atrioventricular block. The latter may be caused by drugs, such as digitalis; myocardial disease, such as myocarditis; myocardial fibrosis related to some type of car-

Table 1   Upper Limits of the Normal PR Intervals

Rate	Below 70	71–90	91–110	111–130	Above 130
Large adults	0.21	0.20	0.19	0.18	0.17
Small adults	0.20	0.19	0.18	0.17	0.16
Children ages 14–17	0.19	0.18	0.17	0.16	0.15
Children ages 7–13	0.18	0.17	0.16	0.15	0.14
Children ages 1½–6	0.17	0.165	0.155	0.145	0.135
Children ages 0–1½	0.16	0.15	0.145	0.135	0.125

From Ashman R, Hull E: *Essentials of electrocardiography*, ed. 2, New York, 1941, Macmillan, p 341. The copyright was transferred to the authors in 1956. The authors are deceased.

diomyopathy or coronary atherosclerotic heart disease; and the aging process, including apoptosis of some of the cells in the AV node and beyond.

The duration of the QRS complex signifies how long it takes the ventricles to depolarize. The duration of the QRS complex in a normal newborn may be 0.06 second and the duration of the QRS complex in a normal adult should be less than 0.10 second. The duration of the QRS complexes may become slightly longer when the ventricles become larger than normal but it is rarely longer than 0.10 second. The duration of the QRS complex becomes considerably longer when the left or right ventricular conduction systems are damaged. At times the duration of the QRS complex may become 0.16 or 0.18 second. This extreme abnormality is commonly due to complicated left or right ventricular conduction system abnormality plus left or right ventricular enlargement.

The duration of the Q-T interval must be determined with great care because it may be prolonged in patients with certain electrolyte abnormalities; in patients taking drugs that produce a serious proarrhythmic state; patients with genetically determined repolarization abnormalities such as those responsible for the long Q-T sudden death syndrome and the Brugada syndrome; and in patients with myocardial disease due to one of several causes.

The duration of the Q-T interval varies with the heart rate. Although there are formulae that can be used to determine the normalcy of the Q-T interval, it is easier to refer to standard tables that relate the duration of the Q-T interval to the heart rate (see Table 12–2). The interpreter should inspect the tracing itself to determine the Q-T interval instead of using the computer readout of the measurement. This is necessary because the reference tables were created before computers were developed.

The greatest problem in the measurement of the Q-T interval is that it is difficult to measure; it is not always easy to identify when the end of the T wave reaches the baseline. In addition, it is useful to determine if the increased length

Table 2 Normal QT Intervals and the Upper Limits of Normal

Cycle lengths (sec)	Heart rate (per min)	Men and children (sec)	Women (sec)	Upper limits of normal — Men and children (sec)	Upper limits of normal — Women (sec)
1.50	40	0.449	0.461	0.491	0.503
1.40	43	0.438	0.450	0.479	0.491
1.30	46	0.426	0.438	0.466	0.478
1.25	48	0.420	0.432	0.460	0.471
1.20	50	0.414	0.425	0.453	0.464
1.15	52	0.407	0.418	0.445	0.456
1.10	54.5	0.400	0.411	0.438	0.449
1.05	57	0.393	0.404	0.430	0.441
1.00	60	0.386	0.396	0.422	0.432
0.95	63	0.378	0.388	0.413	0.423
0.90	66.5	0.370	0.380	0.404	0.414
0.85	70.5	0.361	0.371	0.395	0.405
0.80	75	0.352	0.362	0.384	0.394
0.75	80	0.342	0.352	0.374	0.384
0.70	86	0.332	0.341	0.363	0.372
0.65	92.5	0.321	0.330	0.351	0.360
0.60	100	0.310	0.318	0.338	0.347
0.55	109	0.297	0.305	0.325	0.333
0.50	120	0.283	0.291	0.310	0.317
0.45	133	0.268	0.276	0.294	0.301
0.40	150	0.252	0.258	0.275	0.282
0.35	172	0.234	0.240	0.255	0.262

From Ashman R, Hull E: *Essentials of electrocardiography*, ed 2, New York, 1941, *Macmillan*, p 344. The copyright was transferred to the authors in 1956. The authors are deceased.

of the Q-T interval is due to a longer than normal duration of the QRS complex, S-T segment, or T wave (1).

The "U" wave may join the T wave and produce a long "Q-U" interval. Views have changed during the past few years regarding this phenomenon, which commonly occurs with hypokalemia, because of the new work by Antzelevitch and his coworkers regarding the genesis of what was once called abnormal U waves (2,3). In brief, he no longer labels what we once called abnormal U waves by that name because he and his associates have shown that such waves are actually interrupted T waves. This is why the quotation marks are used in the first sentence of this paragraph; *the waves we once called U waves are not U waves.* This is discussed later in this chapter under the heading of *U waves.*

There are no tables that indicate the lower limits of the normal Q-T interval. The Q-T interval may be short in patients taking digitalis, patients with hypercalcemia, and for unexplained reasons. The Q-T interval represents the amount of time required for the ventricles to depolarize, plus the amount of time in which no electrical forces are produced, plus the amount of time required for the ventricles to repolarize. Apparently some individuals with a short Q-T interval are simply able to repolarize their myocytes earlier than other people. This seems to cause an increase in the lability of the T waves because they change more than usual with a change in posture. This phenomenon appears to be unimportant except that the finding may be misinterpreted. The inherently short Q-T interval has been studied very little, but the condition makes one wonder if there might be a currently unrecognized complication of such a finding. We know there is a long Q-T interval syndrome and it is reasonable to consider the possibility that there might be a short Q-T interval syndrome. In addition, it makes sense to look for possible arrhythmias when there is any alteration in the time required for repolarization.

Characteristics of the Normal P, and Ta Waves,
QRS Complexes, S-T Segments, and T Waves

P Waves

The amplitude of the P waves of normal adults is less than 2.5 millimeters and the duration of the normal P waves is about 0.10 second.

The mean P wave vector is normally directed at about +50° inferiorly and is parallel with the frontal plane or directed only slightly anteriorly. When there is lower atrial rhythm the mean P vector is directed superiorly and to the left.

The mean vector representing the first half of the normal P wave, which is produced by depolarization of the right atrium, is normally directed at about +50° in the frontal plane and about 10° anteriorly (Fig. 7-1). When the P wave is somewhat pointed and is greater than 2.5 mm high in lead II, or in any of the extremity leads, a *right atrial abnormality* is said to be present. In such cases the first half of the P wave is usually prominent in lead V_1. When the P waves are large, as described above, and the mean P vector is directed 70° or more to the right and anteriorly, the interpreter should look for cor pulmonale due to obstructive lung disease and emphysema. A right atrial abnormality *suggests an abnormality of the right ventricle or tricuspid valve disease.*

The normal mean vector representing the last half of the normal P wave, which is produced by depolarization of the left atrium, is usually directed at about +40° to +50° in the frontal plane and is directed about 10° to 15° posteriorly (see Fig. 7-1). Note that the normal mean vector for the second half of the P wave is directed slightly posterior to the mean vector representing the first half of the P wave. The size of the vector representing the second half of the P wave should be determined as follows. The second half of the normal P wave in lead V_1 should be less than 0.04 second in duration and less than 1 millimeter deep. The total area of the second half of the normal P wave in lead V_1 should be less than −0.04 mm/sec (4). The second half of the normal P wave is uncommonly inverted in lead V_2. When the duration of the P wave is 0.12 second and notched in the middle, the second half of the P wave is isoelectric or negative in lead V_2, and the area of the second half of the P wave in lead V_1 is greater than −0.04 mm/second, a left atrial abnormality is usually present. *This signifies an abnormality of the left ventricle or mitral valve.*

The word *abnormality* is used to identify the deviations from normal observed in the P waves because the abnormali-

ties are not always related to dilatation or the atria; most of
the abnormalities are probably due to conduction defects in
the atria. There is no evidence that atrial hypertrophy is the
cause of P wave abnormalities and such a designation is
clearly wrong.

Ta Waves

The repolarization of the atria produces a small vector that
is directed opposite to the direction of the mean P vector.
This is referred to as the T of the P (see Fig. 7-2). It cannot
be seen in all leads and its spatial orientation usually cannot
be determined. The T of the P (Ta) may be seen when the P-
R interval is at the upper limit of the normal range or is long,
and it may occasionally be seen during the S-T segment when
the P-R interval is short. Other causes of a prominent displacement of the P-R interval are pericarditis and atrial infarction.

QRS Complexes

The characteristics of normal QRS complexes are as follows:
The *duration of normal QRS complexes* in the adult is
less than 0.10 second.
The *direction of the normal mean QRS vector* varies with
age. The mean QRS vector is directed to the right and anteriorly in the normal newborn (see Fig. 12-1A). This is to be expected because the right ventricle of the newborn child is as
thick or thicker than the left ventricle. After birth the pulmonary arterial resistance decreases and the peripheral arterial
resistance increases, causing the gradual increase in thickness of the left ventricle as compared to the thickness of the
right ventricle. This causes the mean QRS vector to shift gradually to the left and posteriorly. The direction of the mean QRS
vector is determined by the location and thickness of the two
ventricles; the direction of the mean vector being the vector
sum of the vectors produced by each of the two ventricles. Accordingly, the mean QRS vector is directed more vertically and

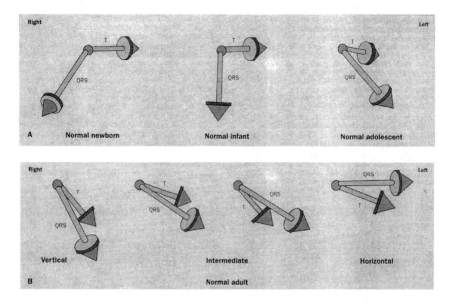

Figure 12-1 *A.* The figure to the left shows the direction of the mean QRS vector and mean T vector in a normal newborn. Note the mean QRS vector is directed to the right and anteriorly because electrical forces produced by depolarization of the right ventricle, which is located to the right of the left ventricle and anteriorly, dominates the electrical field. The figures in the middle and to the right show the direction of the mean QRS vector and mean T vector in a normal infant and adolescent. Note, as the left ventricle begins to dominate the electrical field, that the mean QRS vector shifts to the left and posteriorly. The mean T vector continues to be directed to the left and posteriorly, but the QRS-T angle becomes less. *B.* This panel of illustrations depicts a normal vertical mean QRS vector, a normal intermediate QRS vector, and a normal horizontal mean QRS vector in adults. The direction of the mean QRS vector is greatly influenced by the body build of the patient; the mean QRS vector is more likely to be directed vertically in a tall person, more horizontally in a broad-chested or obese patient, and intermittently in the person of average build. As shown here, the normal mean T vector is directed to the left of a vertically directed mean QRS vector. The normal mean T vector is directed to the right or left of an intermediate mean QRS vector and inferior to a horizontally directed mean QRS vector. The mean T vector is always directed anterior to the mean QRS vector and the QRS-T angle is 45° to 60°. (*Source:* Hurst JW. *Ventricular Electrocardiography*. New York: Gower Medical Publishing, 1991:5–16. The author, J.W.H., owns the copyright.)

parallel with the frontal plane in the older child and adolescent (see Fig. 12-1A).

The direction of the mean QRS vector in adults varies with the body build (see Fig. 12-1). The tall person usually has a more *vertical positioned heart* and the broad-chested person usually has a more *horizontally positioned heart*. The hearts of most people are located in between the *vertical* and *horizontal* position and their hearts are referred to as being in an *intermediate* position. The vector representing the direction of depolarization of the ventricles is influenced by the anatomic position of the heart, the thickness of the ventricles, and the function of the conduction system of both ventricles. Accordingly, the direction of the normal mean QRS vector in adults may be located from about $+90°$ to $+100°$ to about $-20°$ to $-30°$ in the frontal plane and from $35°$ to $50°$ posteriorly. The mean QRS vectors in *most* adults is directed at $+30°$ to $+60°$ in the frontal plane and about $45°$ posteriorly. As discussed earlier, when the mean QRS vector is directed toward the numbers located at the edges of the distribution curve, say at $+90°$ or $-20°$ in the frontal plane, the finding is not normal 100 percent of the time. This is true because abnormal findings overlap the normal finding at the edges of the distribution curve. The directions of mean QRS vectors in normal adults are shown in Figure 12–1B.

The *amplitude of the QRS* complexes must be measured. Each generation of investigators has tried to define the normal amplitude of the QRS complexes. This, of course, is not really possible, because the electrical potential recorded from surface electrodes is influenced by the shape of the chest and the amount of chest musculature and adipose tissue, which varies from person to person. The latest criteria are those developed by Odom (5) and Siegel (6) and their coworkers (5). They suggest that the normal range of 12-lead QRS amplitude in adults is about 80 to 185 millimeters. This measurement is determined by adding arithmetically the depth of the Q waves to the height of the R waves to the depth of the S waves in all

12 leads. Like all normal ranges, the edges of the range are overlapped by the abnormal.

A 12-lead QRS amplitude that is 190 millimeters in adults may suggest the presence of left ventricular hypertrophy due to one of various causes when the QRS duration is 0.10 second or less in duration and when the mean QRS vector is directed inferiorly to the left and posteriorly. As expected, a QRS amplitude located at the upper end of the normal range, say 170 millimeters, may be abnormal in a certain number of instances. Remember, only the measurements located in the middle part of a normal distribution curve are always normal; abnormal measurements overlap the normal measurements at the edges of the distribution curve. As discussed in Chapter 13, if the only abnormality is a greater-than-normal 12-lead QRS amplitude of the QRS complexes, it permits only a diagnosis of *probable* left ventricular hypertrophy; other electrocardiographic abnormalities must be present to definitely identify left ventricular hypertrophy. The 12-lead QRS amplitude measurement cannot be used in neonates and young children because they exhibit large amplitude of the QRS complex simply because the surface electrodes are so near the heart.

As will be explained in Chapter 14, a measurement of the amplitude of the mean QRS complexes is usually not needed to diagnose right ventricular hypertrophy.

The identification of the low end of the normal range of QRS amplitude as described by Odom (5) and Seigel (6) is useful because prior to their report, there were few studies that indicated when abnormally low amplitude of the QRS complexes was present. Here, too, abnormally low amplitude of the QRS complexes may overlap the lower edge of the distribution curve for normal QRS amplitude. When low amplitude of the QRS complexes is present, it may be due to improper standardization of the electrocardiograph machine, pericardial effusion, dilated cardiomyopathy, obesity, myxedema, scleroderma, anasarca, or emphysema.

The mean vector representing the electrical forces that produce the *initial 0.04 second of the QRS complex in normal adults* has a special relationship with the mean QRS vector (see Fig. 12–2). The mean initial 0.04 second QRS vector in normal adults should be directed to the left of a vertical mean QRS vector, on either side of an intermediate mean QRS vector and inferior to a horizontal mean QRS vector. The initial mean 0.04 second QRS vector is always anterior to the mean spatial QRS vector and the normal angle between the two is usually 45° to 60°.

The direction of this vector and its relationship to the mean QRS vector is used to identify myocardial infarction. Parenthetically, it should be emphasized that in some patients the mean initial 0.02 second vector may become abnormal secondary to myocardial infarction and that abnormal initial

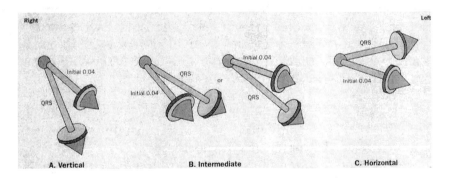

Figure 12-2 This figure shows the direction of the mean electrical forces generated during the initial 0.04 second of the QRS complex. Note that the normal mean initial 0.04 second vector is directed to the left of a vertical mean QRS vector, on either side of an intermediate mean QRS vector, and inferior to a normal mean QRS vector. It is always anterior to the mean QRS vector and the angle between the mean initial 0.04 second vector and the mean QRS vector is about 45° to 60°. (*Source:* Hurst JW. *Ventricular Electrocardiography.* New York: Gower Medical Publishing, 1991:5–18. The author, J.W.H., owns the copyright.)

QRS forces may be caused by conditions other than myocardial infarction.

The mean vector representing the electrical forces that produce the *terminal 0.04 second of the QRS complex in normal adults* is shown in Figure 12–3. Note the relationship of the mean terminal 0.04 vector to the mean QRS vector as shown in figure 12–3. The direction of the terminal 0.04 vector is always located posterior to the mean QRS vector. It is commonly directed to the right of a vertical mean QRS vector, either side of an intermediate QRS vector, and superior to a horizontal QRS vector. This vector, as well as the vector representing the electrical forces that produce the last 0.02 second of the QRS complex, is used to identify right and left ventricular conduction system abnormalities.

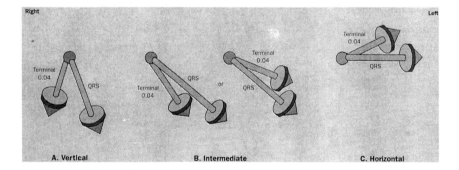

Figure 12-3   This figure shows the direction of the mean electrical forces generated during the last 0.04 second of the QRS complex. The mean terminal 0.04 second vector is usually directed to the right of the mean vertical QRS vector, on either side of the intermediate QRS vector, and usually superior to the horizontal QRS vector. The terminal 0.04 second QRS vector is always posterior to the mean QRS vector and the angle between the mean terminal 0.04 second vector and the mean QRS vector is about 45° to 60°. (*Source*: Hurst JW. *Ventricular Electrocardiography*. New York: Gower Medical Publishing, 1991:5–16. The author, J.W.H., owns the copyright.)

S-T Segment

The normal S-T segment is usually not displaced upward or downward from the baseline which is determined by comparing its location to the location of the line creating the T-P interval. A mean S-T vector may be seen in a small percentage of normal subjects; it is seen more commonly in young people. The vector representing the mean S-T segment displacement in such cases is directed parallel with a large, but normally directed mean T wave vector. Such an S-T segment displacement is caused by early repolarization of the ventricles and is actually part of the large T wave. The repolarization process is controlled by certain genes. The repolarization process simply begins earlier in some normal people than it does in other normal people. The tracings that exhibit this normal finding are referred to as showing "early repolarization" (see Fig. 12–4).

The S-T segment may be abnormally displaced because of a large number of different causes, including left and right ventricular hypertrophy, left and right conduction system block, epicardial and endocardial injury, pericarditis, digitalis

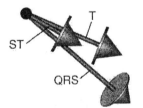

Figure 12-4 Early repolarization of the ventricles. Note that the mean S-T vector is parallel with the mean T vector, which is usually larger than normal. This may be normal but it may also occur secondary to diastolic overload of the left ventricle as well as endocardial ischemia. (*Source*: Hurst JW. *Cardiovascular Diagnosis. The Initial Examination*. St. Louis: Mosby-Year Book, Inc, 1993:260. The author, J.W.H., owns the copyright.)

effect, etc. The abnormal S-T vectors responsible for the abnormal deflections are discussed in the chapters that follow.

Normal Mean T Wave Vector

The T wave is produced by repolarization of the ventricles. Although the amplitude of the T wave is not as great as the amplitude of the QRS complex, the T wave is broader than the QRS complex. Theoretically, there should be as much area under the T wave as there is under the QRS complex. In fact, that is usually not the case. The areas are not equal because some of the forces of one of the waves are directed in opposite directions and cancel themselves out.

The T wave is produced late in mechanical systole of the ventricles, whereas the QRS complex initiates mechanical systole. This sentence should be read again because many people erroneously believe that the T wave is produced during mechanical diastole. The physiological environment associated with repolarization is quite different from the physiological environment produced by depolarization of the ventricles. As discussed earlier, the repolarization process should *theoretically* be directed from endocardium to epicardium. It should follow the path created by depolarization that proceeds from endocardium to epicardium if the time interval between the loss of electrical charges and the rebuilding of electrical charges is the same throughout the ventricular myocardium. Should this occur, the mean T vector would be directed opposite to the direction of the mean QRS vector. If this sentence is not understood, the reader should review Chapter 4 of this book. *In reality* the repolarization process of the ventricles in a normal adult begins at the epicardium and proceeds toward the endocardium. This implies that the delay in repolarization is greater at the endocardium than the epicardium. The reason for this is not absolutely clear but Grant believed that the transmyocardial pressure gradient plays a major role in reversing the direction of the repolarization process (7). The systolic ventricular pressure is greater in the endocardium than it is in the epicardium. This is believed to be the cause of the delay in repolarization of the endocardium that causes the reversal of the repolarization process. To repeat, the repolarization process is directed from epicardium to endocardium, producing an electrical force that is directed from endocardium to epicardium (see Fig. 7-4). This, of course, would produce a mean T vector that is relatively parallel with the mean QRS vector. Parenthetically, it is useful to consider the many ways the repolarization process could be altered by considering physiological or pathological conditions such as high and low systolic ventricular pressure, ischemia of the epicardium or endocardium, and the effect of drugs that alter the myocardium; these conditions could enhance, diminish, or change the direction of the mean T vector.

Despite the fact that the direction of the normal repolarization process in human ventricles differs from that discussed in the theoretical state, the direction of the wave of repolarization in the human is predetermined by the direction of the depolarization process. Accordingly, an "interpreter" of electrocardiograms should not judge the normality of T waves independent of their relationship with the QRS complexes.

The mean T vector of the normal newborn is directed almost opposite to the mean QRS vector (see Fig. 12-1A). The mean QRS vector is directed to the right and anteriorly, where the dominant right ventricle of the normal neonate is located, and the mean T vector is directed in an opposite direction. The mean T vector is directed away from the right ventricle because the right ventricle is thick as the result of the elevated right ventricular pressure that existed during fetal life. When the first breath is taken, the pulmonary arterial resistance falls and the right ventricular pressure decreases, but the right ventricle remains thick. This causes the transmyocardial pressure gradient in the right ventricle to decrease. This theoretically would permit the repolarization process to begin in the endocardium and produce a T vector that tends to be directed away from the right ventricle. The mean T wave vector may not be directed precisely opposite to the direction of the mean vector representing the QRS complexes because the direction of the mean T vector is produced by the summation of the direction of repolarization forces produced by the right ventricle plus those produced by the left ventricle.

The anatomic and physiological conditions that are present at birth gradually change: The pulmonary arterial resistance falls and the peripheral arterial resistance increases as the months pass and eventually the left ventricle is thicker than the right ventricle. During childhood and adolescence the mean QRS vector shifts toward the left and posteriorly and the mean T vector shifts to the left and inferiorly but retains its posterior direction until the teenage period (see Fig. 12-1A).

The direction of the normal mean T vector of the adult has a locked-in relationship to the direction of the mean QRS vector. The normal mean T vector should be located to the left of a *vertically* directed normal mean QRS vector (see Fig. 12-1B). It is always anterior to the mean QRS vector and the spatial angle between the two vectors is 45° to 60°. The normal mean T vector may be directed to the right or left of an *intermediately* directed mean QRS vector. It must be directed anterior to the mean QRS vector and the QRS-T spatial angle is 45° to 60°. The normal mean T vector should be located inferior to a *horizontally* directed mean QRS vector. It is always anterior to the mean QRS vector and the spatial angle between the two is 45° to 60°.

The mean vectors representing the twelve QRS complexes and the twelve T waves should be drawn according to their size. For example, if the area under the QRS complexes is the same as the area under the T wave, the vectors representing each of them should be drawn to be equal in length. When the area under the T waves is smaller or larger than the area under the QRS complexes, the length of the mean T vector should be adjusted accordingly. When the foregoing is accomplished, it is possible to calculate the direction of the *ventricular gradient* (8). The ventricular gradient can be estimated by creating a parallelagram using the mean QRS vector as one side and the mean T vector as the other side; the diagonal becomes the ventricular gradient. The ventricular gradient in the adult should be directed inferiorly and to the left. It should be longer than the mean QRS and T vectors and its terminus should be in the left lower quadrant of the hexaxial reference system (between 0° and +90°). Its anteroposterior position should be between the mean QRS and mean T vectors. The ventricular gradient is a measure of the extent to which repolarization follows the dictates of depolarization. Its calculation is useful, as will be discussed later, in separating the *secondary T wave abnormalities* that accompany left and right ventricular conduction system abnormalities from *primary T wave abnormalities* due to other causes that may be seen when such QRS conduction defects are present.

T wave abnormalities are caused by a diverse group of cardiac conditions. T wave alternans is abnormal and may be a precursor of ventricular arrhythmias, including torsade de pointes (9). The conditions responsible for T wave abnormalities will be discussed in the chapters that follow.

U Waves

U waves may not be seen in normal electrocardiograms. When they are seen, they are not seen in all leads and cannot be converted to a single mean vector. There are no measurements available that delineate the size of normal U waves. A rough approach to this problem is to assume that normal U waves are about one-fourth the size of the T waves that are associated with them. *Normal U waves are caused by the repolarization of the His-Purkinje system.*

Abnormal U waves are large or inverted. Inverted U waves are virtually always associated with conditions such as hypokalemia, hypertension, coronary atherosclerotic heart disease, advanced valve disease, or cardiomyopathy (10). The same is probably true for abnormally large U waves. According to Antzelevitch and his coworkers, abnormally large or inverted U waves are not the result of the repolarization of the His-Purkinje system (2,3). There is simply not a sufficient amount of such tissue to produce large U waves. The deflections that we formerly called abnormal U waves should not be called U waves according to Antzelevitch; they are interrupted or split T waves (2,3). The M cells, identified by Antzelevitch et al., which look like other myocytes but function somewhat differently, lie near the middle of the left ventricular muscle and normally do not alter the course of repolarization. When the left ventricle is diseased, the M cells participate by interrupting the wave of repolarization. Two separate repolarization vectors are produced. The second one was formerly called the U wave, but it is really the second part of the T wave.

Waves Other than the P Wave, QRS Complex, and U Waves

The T of the P must be sought. The repolarization wave of the atria (Ta wave) occurs after the P wave and the vector that represents it is directed opposite to the vector that represents the P wave. The normal Ta wave must be differentiated from the P-Q segment displacement due to acute pericarditis. The T of the P may also cause the S-T segment to be slightly displaced when the P-R interval is short and must not be mistaken for an abnormally displaced S-T segment.

The delta wave is the term applied to the slurred initial portion of the QRS complex that is caused by preexcitation of the ventricles (2). Patients with this condition have a short P-R interval and a prolonged duration of the QRS complex. As discussed in Chapter 23, such an abnormality may be responsible for paroxysmal atrial tachycardia or paroxysmal atrial fibrillation (Wolff-Parkinson-White syndrome).

The Osborn wave is usually caused by hypothermia (2). This type of postexcitation of the ventricles is discussed in Chapter 23. The Osborn wave is sometimes called a camel-hump located in the descending portion of the QRS complex.

The S-T segments in leads V_1-V_3 must be studied in an effort to observe epsilon waves (see Chapter 23). These waves were initially described by Fontaine and occur in patients with post excitation of the right ventricle due to right ventricular dysplasia (2). Other diseases in which islands of myocytes within the right ventricular wall are surrounded by "inert" tissue may also produce the substrate necessary for the produc-

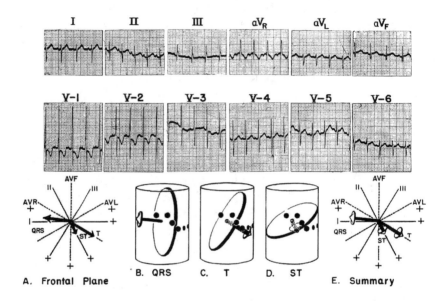

Figure 12-5 This electrocardiogram was recorded from a 2-day-old normal infant. There are 160 complexes per minute. The duration of the QRS complexes is 0.06 second. Note the large amplitude of the QRS complexes. The mean QRS vector is directed to the right (at −170°) in the frontal plane and anteriorly about 40°. The mean T vector is directed at +30° in the frontal plane and about 20° posteriorly. The spatial QRS-T angle is about 170°. The mean S-T vector is directed about 45° from the mean T vector. This is a normal electrocardiogram. See text for further discussion. (*Source*: Hurst JW, Woodson GC Jr. *Atlas of Spatial Vector Electrocardiography*. New York: The Blakiston Company, Inc, 1952:51. The author, J.W.H., owns the copyright.)

tion of epsilon waves. Accordingly, epsilon waves have been observed in right ventricular infarction, right ventricular fibrosis such as occurs with sickle cell anemia, and rarely dilated cardiomyopathy of both ventricles (2).

Brugada waves are seen in the leads V_1-V_3 in some patients with right bundle branch block (2). These noncoronary

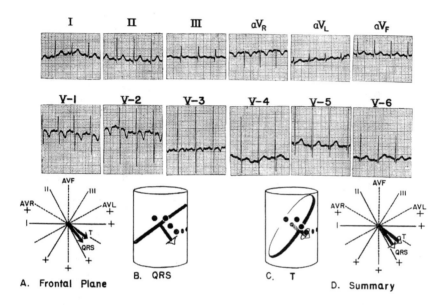

Figure 12-6 This electrocardiogram was recorded from a normal 2-year-old child. There are about 130 complexes per minute. The duration of the QRS complexes is about 0.07 second. Note the large amplitude of the QRS complexes. The mean QRS vector is directed at about +50° in the frontal plane and is almost parallel with the frontal plane. Note that the direction of the mean QRS vector varies slightly, undoubtedly due to inspiration and expiration. The mean T vector is directed at +40° in the frontal plane and about 20° posteriorly. The spatial QRS-T angle is about 15° to 20°. This is a normal electrocardiogram. See text for further discussion. (*Source*: Hurst JW, Woodson GC Jr. *Atlas of Spatial Vector Electrocardiography*. New York: The Blakiston Company, Inc, 1952:53. The author, J.W.H., owns the copyright.)

S-T segments are caused by abnormal repolarization of a portion of the right ventricle and are associated with arrhythmias and sudden death (11). The mechanism responsible for these noncoronary S-T segments is now under intense study and there is definite evidence that the repolarization abnormality of the Brugada syndrome is genetically determined (see Chapter 23).

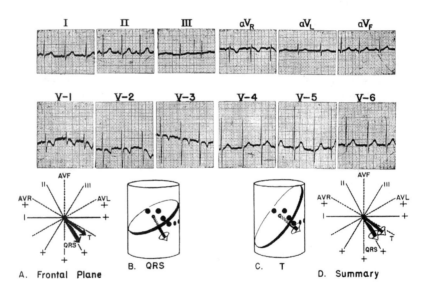

A. Frontal Plane   B. QRS   C. T   D. Summary

Figure 12-7 This electrocardiogram was recorded from a normal 3½-year-old child. There are 150 complexes per minute. The duration of the QRS complex is 0.07 second. The mean QRS vector is directed about 55° in the frontal plane and about 30° posteriorly. The mean T vector is directed about 40° in the frontal plane and about 30° posteriorly. This is a normal electrocardiogram. See text for further discussion. (*Source*: Hurst JW, Woodson GC Jr: Atlas of Spatial Vector Electrocardiography. New York: The Blakiston Company, Inc, 1952:55. The author, J.W.H., owns the copyright.)

EXAMPLES OF NORMAL ELECTROCARDIOGRAMS

The electrocardiogram of a normal 2-day-old neonate is shown in Figure 12-5.

The electrocardiogram of a normal 2-year-old child is shown in Figure 12-6.

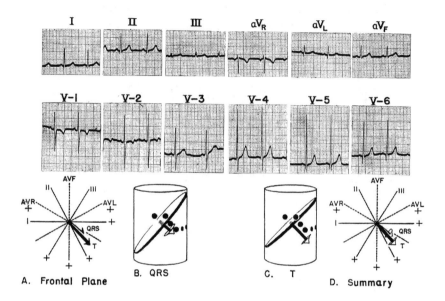

Figure 12-8 This electrocardiogram was recorded from a normal 6-year-old child. There are 90 complexes per minute. The duration of the QRS complexes is about 0.07 second. Note the large QRS amplitude. The mean QRS vector is directed about 35° in the frontal plane and about 15° posteriorly. The mean T vector is directed about 45° in the frontal plane and about 15° posteriorly. The spatial QRS-T angle is 5° to 10°. Note the area subtended by the T wave is larger than the area subtended by the QRS complex. This is a normal electrocardiogram. See text for further discussion. (*Source*: Hurst JW, Woodson GC Jr. *Atlas of Spatial Vector Electrocardiography*. New York: The Blakiston Company, Inc, 1952:57. The author, J.W.H., owns the copyright.)

The electrocardiogram of a normal 3½-year-old child is shown in Figure 12-7.

The electrocardiogram of a normal 6-year-old child is shown in Figure 12-8.

The electrocardiogram of a normal 12-year-old child is shown in Figure 12-9.

The electrocardiogram of an 18-year-old normal subject is shown in Figure 12-10.

This series of tracings illustrates how the mean QRS vector gradually shifts from being directed to the right and anteri-

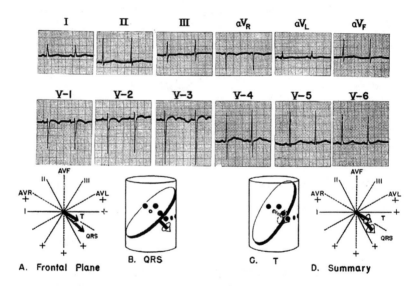

Figure 12-9 This electrocardiogram was recorded from a normal 12-year-old child. There are about 75 complexes per minute. The duration of the QRS complex is 0.07 second. Note the large QRS amplitude. The mean QRS vector is directed about 40° in the frontal plane and about 35° to 40° posteriorly. The mean T vector is directed about 25° to 30° in the frontal plane and 35° to 40° posteriorly. This is a normal electrocardiogram. See text for further discussion. (*Source*: Hurst JW, Woodson GC Jr. *Atlas of Spatial Vector Electrocardiography*. New York: The Blakiston Company, Inc, 1952:59. The author, J.W.H., owns the copyright.)

orly to being directed to the left and posteriorly. The mean T vector shifts from being posteriorly directed to being parallel with the frontal plane or slightly anteriorly directed. The QRS-T angle changes from being about 170° to about 45° or less.

The electrocardiogram of a normal adult whose heart is located vertically is shown in Figure 12-11.

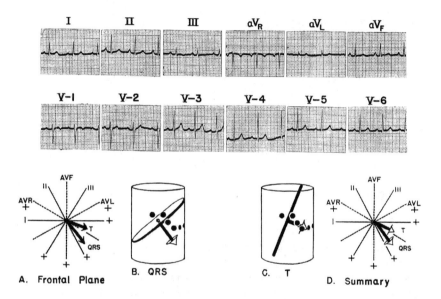

Figure 12-10 This electrocardiogram was recorded from a normal subject, age 18. There are about 87 complexes per minute. The mean QRS vector is directed about +50° in the frontal plane and about 15° posteriorly. The mean T vector is directed about +20° in the frontal plane and is parallel with the frontal plane. The QRS-T angle is about 25°–30°. Note the T_A waves in leads II and V_2 and the small normal U wave in lead V_2. The elevated S-T segment, seen best in lead V_4, is due to normal early repolarization. This is a normal electrocardiogram. See text for further discussion. (*Source*: Hurst JW, Woodson GC Jr. *Atlas of Spatial Vector Electrocardiography*. New York: The Blakiston Company, Inc, 1952:61. The author, J.W.H., owns the copyright.)

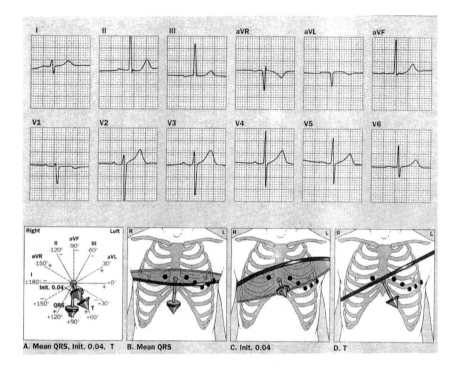

Figure 12-11 This electrocardiogram was recorded from a 37-year-old normal, tall, thin, male. The duration of the QRS is 0.08 second. The direction of the mean QRS vector is about +90° in the frontal plane and 40° posteriorly. The direction of the mean T vector is about +70° in the frontal plane; it is parallel with the frontal plane. The QRS-T angle is about 20°. The mean 0.04 second QRS vector is directed about 70° in the frontal plane and at least 20° to 30° anteriorly. This is an example of a vertical mean QRS vector. This electrocardiogram is normal. (*Source:* Upper portion from Hurst JW. *Ventricular Electrocardiography.* New York: Gower Medical Publishing, 1991:5.25. The author, J.W.H., owns the copyright. Lower portion from Hurst JW. *Cardiovascular Diagnosis. The Initial Examination.* St. Louis: Mosby-Year Book, Inc, 1993:262. The author, J.W.H., owns the copyright.)

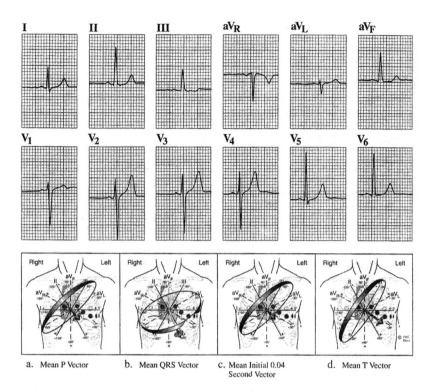

a. Mean P Vector   b. Mean QRS Vector   c. Mean Initial 0.04   d. Mean T Vector
                                           Second Vector

Figure 12-12 This electrocardiogram was recorded from a 27-year-old man of average build. The duration of the QRS complexes is 0.08 second. The direction of the mean QRS complex is +70° in the frontal plane and about 50° posteriorly. The direction of the mean T vector is +35° in the frontal plane and about 30° anteriorly. The QRS-T angle is about 35°. The direction of the initial mean 0.04 second QRS vector is about +55° in the frontal plane and about 30° anteriorly. This is an example of an intermediate mean QRS vector. This electrocardiogram is normal. (*Source*: Upper portion from Hurst JW. *Ventricular Electrocardiography*. New York: Gower Medical Publishing, 1991:5.26. The author, J.W.H., holds the copyright. Lower portion from Hurst JW. *Cardiovascular Diagnosis. The Initial Examination*. St. Louis: Mosby-Year Book, Inc, 1993:264. The author, J.W.H., owns the copyright.)

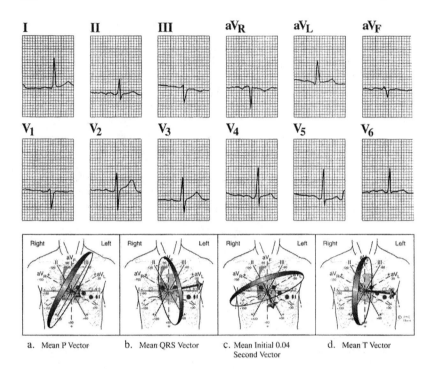

a. Mean P Vector   b. Mean QRS Vector   c. Mean Initial 0.04 Second Vector   d. Mean T Vector

Figure 12-13 This electrocardiogram was recorded from a 31-year-old, normal, broad-chested, obese male. The mean QRS vector is directed about $-10°$ to the left in the frontal plane about $15°$ posteriorly. The mean T vector is directed about $+5°$ in the frontal plane and about $10°$ anteriorly. The spatial QRS-T angle is about $15°$. The QRS-T angle is about $25°$. The mean 0.04 second QRS vector is directed about $+70°$ in the frontal plane and at least $20°$ anteriorly. This is an example of a horizontal mean QRS vector. This electrocardiogram is normal. (*Source*: Upper portion from Hurst JW. *Ventricular Electrocardiography*. New York: Gower Medical Publishing, 1991:5.27. The author, J.W.H., owns the copyright. Lower portion from Hurst JW. *Cardiovascular Diagnosis. The Initial Examination*. St. Louis: Mosby-Year Book, Inc, 1993:266. The author, J.W.H., owns the copyright.)

The electrocardiogram of a normal adult whose heart is located in the intermediate position is shown in Figure 12-12. The electrocardiogram of a normal adult whose heart is located in the horizontal position is shown in Figure 12-13.

REFERENCES

1. Hurst JW. Abnormalities of the S-T segment—Part I & Part II. Clin Cardiol 1997; 20:511–520, 595–600.

2. Hurst JW. Naming of the waves in the ECG, with a brief account of their genesis. Circulation 1998;98:1937–1942.

3. Antzelevitch C. The M cell. J Cardiovasc Pharmacol Ther 1997; 2:73–76.

4. Morris JJ, Estes EH Jr, Whalen RE et al. P wave analysis in valvular heart disease. Circulation 1964;29:242.

5. Odom H II, Davis JL, Dinh HA, et al. QRS voltage measurements in autopsied men free of cardiopulmonary disease: a basis for evaluating total QRS voltage as an index of left ventricular hypertrophy. Am J Cardiol 1986;58:801.

6. Siegel RJ, Roberts WC. Electrocardiographic observations in severe aortic valve stenosis: correlative necropsy study to clinical, hemodynamic, and ECG variables demonstrating relation of 12-lead QRS amplitude to peak systolic transaortic pressure gradient. Am Heart J 1982;103:212.

7. Grant RP. *Clinical Electrocardiography*. New York: The Blakiston Division, McGraw-Hill Book Company, Inc, 1957:69.

8. Burch G, Winsor T. *A Primer of Electrocardiography*. Philadelphia: Lea & Febiger, 1945;186.

9. Surawicz B. *Electrophysiologic Basis of ECG and Cardiac Arrhythmias*. Baltimore: Williams & Wilkins, 1995:156–157.

10. Surawicz B. *Electrophysiologic Basis of ECG and Cardiac Arrhythmias*. Baltimore: Williams & Wilkins, 1995:598–599.

11. Bezzina C, Veldkamp MW, van den Berg MP, et al. A single Na+ channel mutation casuing both long-QT and Brugada syndromes. Circ Res 1999;85:1206–1213.

Part VI

Common Electrocardiographic
Abnormalities

Chapter 13

Left Ventricular Hypertrophy

The left ventricular myocardium responds differently to systolic pressure overload of the left ventricle than it does to diastolic pressure overload of the left ventricle (1,2). Systolic pressure overload leads to left ventricular hypertrophy with *little dilatation* of the left ventricular cavity, whereas diastolic pressure overload leads to left ventricular hypertrophy with *considerable dilatation* of the left ventricle.

LEFT VENTRICULAR HYPERTROPHY DUE TO SYSTOLIC PRESSURE OVERLOAD OF THE LEFT VENTRICLE

There are three major electrocardiographic signs of left ventricular hypertrophy due to systolic pressure overload of the left ventricle. They are as follows:

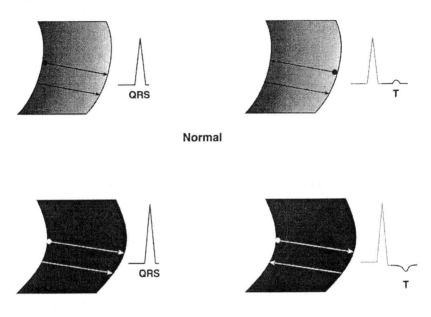

Normal

**Left ventricular hypertrophy due to systolic
pressure overload of the left ventricle**

Figure 13-1   This figure illustrates one theory that attempts to explain some of the electrocardiographic abnormalities associated with systolic pressure overload of the left ventricle. *Top*: The production of the normal QRS and T waves. The shading of the ventricular muscle indicates that the myocardial pressure is greater in the endocardium than it is at the epicardium. This produces a transmyocardial pressure gradient. The creation of the QRS complex is shown to the reader's left. Note that the direction of the depolarization *process* is illustrated by the arrow •→ and that it produces an electrical *force* that is directed in the same direction (illustrated by arrow →). The transmyocardial pressure gradient is produced by ventricular contraction that is *initiated* by the depolarization process. Therefore, the direction of the electrical force is from endocardium to epicardium. This produces an upright QRS complex.

The production of the normal T wave is shown to the reader's right. The shading of the ventricular muscle illustrates that the myocardial pressure is greater at the endocardium than the epicardi-

Left Atrial Abnormality

A left atrial abnormality is commonly present. The amplitude of the P wave is less than 2.5 mm, but the duration of the P wave may be 0.12 second, which is a little longer than usual. The mean P wave vector is usually directed at about +50° in the frontal plane and is parallel with the frontal plane or di-

---

um. This produces a transmyocardial pressure gradient. As discussed above, the depolarization process stimulates the myocytes to contract and produce the transmyocardial pressure gradient. Accordingly, the transmyocardial pressure gradient is just beginning to develop when the QRS complex is produced. On the other hand, *a greater transmyocardial pressure gradient is well established* when the T wave is produced. Therefore, the repolarization *process* is directed from the epicardium toward the endocardium as illustrated by the arrow ←•. This produces an electrical *force* that is opposite to the direction of the process. The direction of the electrical forces is illustrated by the arrow →. This produces the upright T wave that is seen normally. *Bottom*: The production of the abnormal QRS and T waves observed in patients with left ventricular hypertrophy due to systolic pressure overload of the left ventricle. Note that the left ventricular myocardium is thicker than was shown in the top illustration. The shading of the muscle indicates that the transmyocardial *pressure gradient* is nonexistent although the intraventricular pressure is greatly elevated. It is thought that the high systolic pressure within the left ventricle creates high intramyocardial pressure that is equally high at the endocardium and the epicardium and that the pressure *gradient* itself becomes much less. The transmyocardial pressure is *created as the QRS complex is formed*. The QRS complex becomes larger because the left ventricular mass is larger, but the direction of the vector representing the QRS changes no more than 30° to 60°.

The direction of the repolarization process is profoundly altered. The repolarization *process* begins at the endocardium, as illustrated by the arrow •→. The process produces an electrical *force* that is directed in the opposite direction as illustrated by the arrow ←. This creates an inverted T wave and an S-T segment displacement that is part of the T wave.

rected 10° to 20° posteriorly. The mean vector for the last half of the P wave may be directed normally in the frontal plane but is commonly directed more posteriorly than usual; the second half of the P wave is negative in lead V_1 and may be negative in lead V_2. The area contained within the second half of the P wave is more than -0.04 mm/sec or more in lead V_1 (3).

Increased QRS Amplitude

The 12-lead QRS *amplitude* may be 185 millimeters or more and the duration of the QRS complexes is less than 0.10 second. When there are no abnormalities other than increased QRS amplitude, one can only conclude that there is *probable left ventricular hypertrophy (2)*.

The exact *direction* of the mean QRS vector is not useful in identifying left ventricular hypertrophy although it is directed to the left and posteriorly. It can be directed from $+80°$ to $-20°$ in the frontal plane, but it is usually directed from $+30°$ to $+60°$.

Abnormally Directed S-T and T Vectors

The mean T vector may be directed varying degrees away from the mean QRS vector. The QRS-T angle may be 90° to 180°. The mean T vector is always anterior to the mean QRS vector. The T wave abnormality is caused by a decrease in the pressure gradient across the left ventricular myocardium although the transmyocardial pressure itself is increased (see Fig. 13-1). The mean S-T vector is directed relatively parallel to the mean T vector; it is caused by the forces of repolarization. When the mean S-T and T wave vectors are directed 90° to 180° away from the mean QRS vector, systolic pressure overload of the left ventricle should be suspected as occurs with systemic hypertension, aortic valve stenosis, and late in the course of severe aortic regurgitation.

When two of the three abnormalities described above—a left atrial abnormality, an increased QRS amplitude, and S-T and T vectors that are directed 90° to 180° away from the

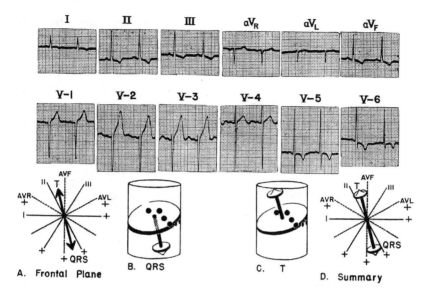

Figure 13-2 This electrocardiogram was recorded from a 32-year-old man with calcific aortic stenosis. The etiology was originally thought to be rheumatic heart disease, but the cause is more likely congenital bicuspid aortic valve stenosis. The duration of the QRS complexes is 0.08 second. The P waves are normal. As shown in A and B, the mean QRS vector is directed at about +75° in the frontal plane and about 50° to 60° posteriorly. The 12-lead QRS amplitude is >254 millimeters (normal upper limit is 185 millimeters).

The mean T vector is directed at about −105° in the frontal plane and about 50° to 60° anteriorly. The QRS-T angle is about 180°. The mean S-T segment vector is parallel to the mean T vector.

The direction and size of the QRS vector and the relationship of the mean T vector to the mean QRS vector are characteristic of systolic pressure overload of the left ventricle. (*Source*: Hurst JW, Woodson GC Jr. *Atlas of Spatial Vector Electrocardiography*. New York: The Blakiston Company, Inc, 1952:89. The author, J.W.H., owns the copyright.)

direction of the mean QRS vector—one can conclude that left ventricular hypertrophy is *definitely present*.

The QRS duration may be 0.10 second and the intrinsicoid deflection of the QRS complexes in leads V_5 or V_6 may be greater than 0.05 second, but these are minor signs of left ventricular hypertrophy.

Occasionally, the entire QRS loop may be rotated posteriorly so that no R waves are seen in leads V_1, V_2 and V_3. Such an abnormality may simulate the initial QRS force abnormality of septal infarction (see discussion in Chapter 15).

An electrocardiogram illustrating systolic pressure overload of the left ventricle is shown in Figure 13-2. The tracing was recorded from a 32-year-old man with severe aortic valve stenosis that was thought to be rheumatic in origin. In retrospect, the aortic valve stenosis was probably due to a congenital bicuspid aortic valve. A similar tracing could be produced by systemic hypertension or idiopathic left ventricular hypertrophy (hypertrophic cardiomyopathy).

LEFT VENTRICULAR HYPERTROPHY DUE TO DIASTOLIC PRESSURE OVERLOAD OF THE LEFT VENTRICLE

Diastolic pressure overload of the left ventricle leads to left ventricular hypertrophy and moderate *dilatation* of the left ventricular cavity.

There are three major signs of left ventricular hypertrophy due to diastolic pressure overload of the left ventricle. They are as follows:

Left Atrial Abnormality

A left atrial abnormality may be present. The reader should review the abnormalities that are characteristic of a left atrial abnormality that are discussed earlier in this chapter.

Increase in QRS Amplitude

There is an increase in 12-lead QRS amplitude; the amplitude may be 185 millimeters or more. The direction of the mean QRS vector may be normal; it may be directed between +80° and −20° in the frontal plane and 30° to 60° posteriorly. The mean vector representing the initial 0.01 to 0.3 second of the QRS complex may be large and directed almost opposite to the direction of the mean QRS vector. This large initial QRS vector is probably produced by the increase in surface area of the endocardium of the dilated left ventricle (including the septum).

The Size and Direction of the S-T and T Vectors

The mean T vector and mean S-T vector are commonly larger than usual and are directed normally during the early stages of left ventricular hypertrophy due to diastolic pressure over-load of the left ventricle. This is probably because the surface area of the endocardium of the left ventricle is greatly in-creased and the volume load that is ejected during systole does not alter the transmyocardial systolic pressure gradient as much as the systolic pressure load produced by aortic valve stenosis or hypertension (see Fig. 13-3). At least this seems to be true during the early stages of diastolic overload of the left ventricle.

When the cause of the diastolic overload of the left ventri-cle is severe as may occur with aortic valve regurgitation, the electrocardiogram may assume the characteristics of systolic pressure overload of the left ventricle including a left atrial abnormality, an increase in the amplitude of the QRS com-plexes, and an S-T and T vector that is directed 90° to 180° away from the direction of the QRS vector.

The QRS duration may be 0.10 second and the duration of the intrinsicoid deflection may be greater than 0.05 second in leads V_5 and V_6, but these are minor signs of left ventricular hypertrophy.

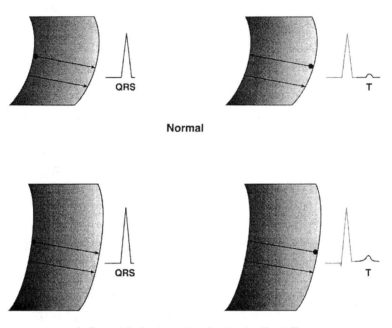

Normal

**Left ventricular hypertrophy due to diastolic
pressure overload of the left ventricle**

Figure 13-3. This figure illustrates one theory that attempts to
explain some of the electrocardiographic abnormalities associated
with diastolic pressure overload of the left ventricle. *Top:* The production of the normal QRS and T waves. The shading of the ventricular muscle indicates that the myocardial pressure is greater in the
endocardium than it is at the epicardium. This produces a transmyocardial pressure gradient. The creation of the QRS complex is shown
to the reader's left. Note that the direction of the depolarization *process* is illustrated by the arrow •→ and that it produces an electrical
force that is directed in the same direction (illustrated by arrow →).
The transmyocardial pressure gradient is produced by ventricular
contraction that is *initiated* by the depolarization process. Therefore,
the direction of the electrical force is from endocardium to epicardium. This produces an upright QRS complex.

The production of the normal T wave is shown to the reader's
right. The shading of the ventricular muscle illustrates that the myocardial pressure is greater at the endocardium than the epicardium.

The vector representing the initial 0.02 to 0.03 second of the QRS complex may be large and, at times, may simulate the abnormal initial QRS vector caused by myocardial infarction (see Chapter 15).

The electrocardiogram shown in Figure 13-4 illustrates diastolic pressure overload of the left ventricle. The tracing was recorded from a 24-year-old man with aortic valve regur-

---

This produces a transmyocardial pressure gradient. As discussed above, the depolarization process stimulates the myocytes to contract and to gradually produce a transmyocardial pressure gradient, whereas a *greater transmyocardial pressure gradient is well established when the T wave is produced.* Accordingly, the repolarization *process* is directed from the epicardium toward the endocardium; it is illustrated by the arrow ←•. The repolarization process produces an electrical *force* that is directed opposite to the direction of the process (illustrated by the arrow →). This produces the upright T wave that is seen normally. *Bottom:* Note that the ventricular muscle is thicker than normal but not as thick as the muscle shown in the bottom illustration of Figure 13-1. Note, too, that the left ventricular cavity is larger than the cavity shown in the bottom illustration of Figure 13-1. The direction of the depolarization *process* is illustrated with the arrow •→. The electrical *force* it produces is illustrated with the arrow →. This produces a larger than normal QRS complex. In some instances the initial 0.04 second QRS vector is also larger than normal and is directed somewhat opposite to the mean QRS vector.

The repolarization process, and the electrical force it produces, are not initially different from normal, because *the transmyocardial pressure gradient is not greatly different from normal.* Note that the shading of the ventricular wall is the same as that shown in the top illustration. The T waves and S-T segments are sometimes larger than normal, presumably because the surface area of the left ventricular cavity is larger than normal. In some instances the initial QRS forces can be confused with the QRS abnormalities of myocardial infarction. When the diastolic pressure is very high, or when diastolic pressure overload has been present a long time, the abnormalities in the tracing become similar to those found in patients with systolic pressure overload of the left ventricle.

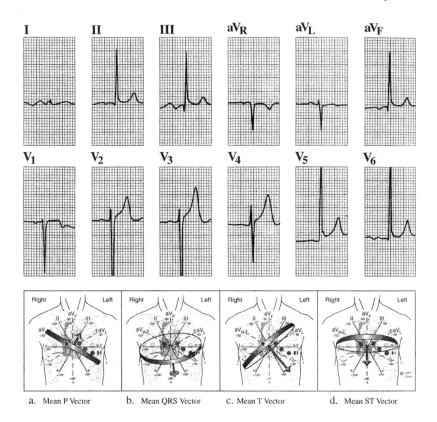

a. Mean P Vector   b. Mean QRS Vector   c. Mean T Vector   d. Mean ST Vector

Figure 13-4   This electrocardiogram was recorded from a 24-year-old man with aortic valve regurgitation due to a congenital bicuspid aortic valve. The P wave vector is abnormal. It is directed superiorly indicating lower atrial rhythm. The QRS duration is 0.08 to 0.09 second. The mean QRS vector is directed at +80° in the frontal plane and about 60° posteriorly. The 12-lead amplitude of the QRS complexes is 230° (upper limit of normal is 185 millimeter). The T waves are larger than usual. The mean T vector is directed at about +50° in the frontal plane and at least 10° anteriorly. The spatial QRS-T angle is about 70°. The mean S-T vector is directed at +90° in the frontal plane and about 10° anteriorly. The S-T—T angle is about 50°, suggesting that the S-T segment displacement is due to repolarization and is therefore part of the T. The direction and size of the QRS vector and the relationship of the S-T and T vectors to the mean

gitation due to a bicuspid aortic valve. A similar tracing could be produced by primary mitral valve regurgitation due to any cause or by aortic valve regurgitation due to any cause, and may be seen in athletes who have diastolic overload of the left ventricle.

ELECTROCARDIOGRAPHIC MYTHS ABOUT LEFT VENTRICULAR HYPERTROPHY

There are several myths about the electrocardiographic signs of left ventricular hypertrophy that must be addressed.

Abnormal "left axis deviation" of the mean QRS vector is not a reliable sign of left ventricular hypertrophy. The direction of the mean QRS vector may shift to the left about 30° from the direction that existed prior to the development of left ventricular hypertrophy; the shift may rarely be as much as 60°. Therefore, "left axis deviation" of the QRS vector is not mentioned as a major sign of left ventricular hypertrophy. Such a finding is commonly caused by left anterior-superior division conduction block. Although left anterior-superior division block can occur in patients with left ventricular hypertrophy, it is not due to hypertrophy.

As mentioned above, when there is no other sign of left ventricular hypertrophy, other than a QRS amplitude that is larger than average, one should label such a tracing as showing *probable* left ventricular hypertrophy. There will never be a magic number of millimeters of QRS amplitude that indicates definite left ventricular hypertrophy. The normal adult heart shows normal left ventricular preponderance and it is

---

QRS vector are characteristic of diastolic pressure overload of the left ventricle. (*Source*: Top: Hurst JW. *Ventricular Electrocardiography*. New York: Gower Medical Publishing, 1991:9.11. The author, JWH, owns the copyright. Bottom: Hurst JW. *Cardiovascular Diagnosis. The Initial Examination*. St. Louis: Mosby-Year Book, Inc, 1993:286. The author, J.W.H, owns the copyright.)

difficult to determine where normal QRS amplitude ends and abnormal QRS amplitude begins. In addition, the amount of adipose tissue and the size of the chest alters the amplitude of the QRS complexes, making it impossible to discover a QRS amplitude that always signifies left ventricular hypertrophy.

The S-T and T wave abnormalities may be difficult to interpret when the patient is taking digitalis.

REFERENCES

1. Cabrera E, Monroy JR. Systolic and diastolic loading of the heart. I. Physiologic and clinical data. Am Heart J 1952;43:661–668.

2. Cabrera E, Monroy JR. Systolic and diastolic loading of the heart. II. Electrocardiographic data. Am Heart J 1952;43:669–686.

3. Morris JJ, Ests EH Jr, Whalen RE, et al. P wave analysis in valvular heart disease. Circulation 1964;29:242–252.

Chapter 14

Right Ventricular Hypertrophy

Right ventricular hypertrophy may be produced by conditions that produce systolic pressure overload of the right ventricle and conditions that produce diastolic overload of the right ventricle (1,2).

RIGHT VENTRICULAR HYPERTROPHY DUE TO SYSTOLIC PRESSURE OVERLOAD OF THE RIGHT VENTRICLE

Right ventricular hypertrophy due to systolic pressure overload of the right ventricle may be caused by *congenital heart disease* such as pulmonary valve stenosis, tetralogy of Fallot, or Eisenmenger syndrome complicating an interventricular septal defect, patent ductus arteriosus, or atrial septal defect. The right ventricular hypertrophy that occurs in patients with Eisenmenger syndrome is similar to acquired causes of right ventricular hypertrophy because initially, patients with interventricular septal defect or patent ductus arteriosus do not have right ventricular hypertrophy; the right ventricular hypertrophy develops after the patients develop pulmonary hypertension due to pulmonary arteriolar disease. Eisenmenger syndrome due to a secundum atrial septal defect is an exception to the rule because such patients may have diastolic pressure overload of the right ventricle before they develop systolic pressure overload of the right ventricle resulting from pulmonary arteriolar disease. Right ventricular hypertrophy due to systolic pressure overload of the right ventricle may also be caused by *acquired diseases* such as lung disease, repeated pulmonary emboli, mitral stenosis, and primary pulmonary hypertension. As discussed below, the electrocardiographic abnormalities produced by congenital heart disease differ from the right ventricular hypertrophy that is produced by acquired heart disease.

Systolic pressure overload of the right ventricle causes the interventricular septum to conform to the circular arrangement of the hypertrophied right ventricle. Accordingly, the electrocardiogram is altered not only because of the thick right ventricle, but also by the new position of the interventricular septum.

Right Ventricular Hypertrophy Persisting from Birth

There are three major signs of right ventricular hypertrophy due to systolic pressure overload of the right ventricle due to congenital heart disease in which the *right ventricular hypertrophy is present from birth* (3). In affected patients, left ventricular dominance never develops.

Right Atrial Abnormality

There may be a right atrial abnormality. The amplitude of the P waves may be greater than 2.5 millimeters. The width of the P wave is usually about 0.10 second. The mean P vector may be normally directed or directed slightly anteriorly. The first half of the P wave in lead V_1 may be larger and more peaked than normal. At times, both right and left atrial abnormalities may be seen because patients with left ventricular disease may develop secondary right ventricular disease and hypertrophy.

Direction of the Mean QRS Vector

The mean QRS vector is directed to the right and anteriorly because the *initial portion* of the QRS complex is large and, when represented as a mean vector, is directed toward the right ventricle. This, of course, may be normal in neonates and in young children. However, the persistence of a mean QRS vector that is directed to the right and anteriorly beyond childhood is abnormal.

There are no 12-lead QRS amplitude criteria for the identification of right ventricular hypertrophy as are used to identify left ventricular hypertrophy. The direction of the mean QRS vector to the right and anteriorly is so obviously different from its direction in normal adults that other criteria are not needed. Accordingly, the direction of the QRS vector is of greater value in establishing the presence of right ventricular hypertrophy than it is in the identification of left ventricular hypertrophy in adults.

Direction of the Mean ST and T Wave Vectors

In adults with right ventricular hypertrophy, the mean S-T and T wave vectors tend to be directed opposite to the direction of the mean QRS vector. They tend to point away from the right ventricle. This occurs because the transmyocardial pressure gradient of the right ventricle is decreased because of the high right ventricular systolic pressure; the pressure at the right ventricular endocardium and epicardium equalizes although it is higher than normal in each of the regions of the right ventricle. This reverses the direction of the electrical forces produced by the repolarization process of the right ventricle. The reader should review Chapter 13 because the same concepts discussed there are operative here.

The mean S-T and T vectors may be directed to the left and anteriorly in the neonate with right ventricular hypertrophy due to systolic pressure overload of the right ventricle. Theoretically, the anterior direction of the S-T and T wave vectors in neonates with right ventricular hypertrophy is related to a right ventricular transmyocardial pressure gradient that permits the repolarization process of the right ventricle to be directed from epicardium to endocardium. This is abnormal because the mean T vector is directed to the left and posteriorly in the normal neonate. This is explained as follows. The transmyocardial pressure gradient in the right ventricle of a normal neonate and child permits the repolarization *process* to be directed from endocardium to epicardium, producing an electrical *force* that is directed in the opposite direction. Presumably, the right ventricular pressure was high prior to birth and the right ventricle was thick. With birth, the pulmonary resistance falls, as does the right ventricular pressure. This leaves a normal, but thick, right ventricle with low right ventricular systolic pressure. This reverses the direction of the repolarization process of the right ventricle in the normal neonate so that repolarization begins in the endocardium of the right ventricle.

The problem in identifying left ventricular hypertrophy in the adult stems from the fact that there is normal left ventricular preponderance in the normal adult. The problem of identifying right ventricular hypertrophy in the neonate and child stems from the fact that there is normal right ventricular preponderance in the normal newborn and young child.

The electrocardiogram shown in Figure 14–1 illustrates systolic pressure overload of the right ventricle in a patient with congenital pulmonary valve stenosis.

Right Ventricular Hypertrophy Occurring After the Development of Left Ventricular Preponderance

There are four major signs of right ventricular hypertrophy that appear *after normal left ventricular preponderance has been established* (3). As stated earlier, acquired causes of right ventricular hypertrophy as well as patients with Eisenmenger syndrome due to interventricular septal defect and patent ductus fall into this group.

Right Atrial Abnormality

Abnormal right atrial P waves may be present. The amplitude of the P waves may be more than 2.5 mm. The mean P vector is directed at about 50° in the frontal plane and anteriorly. The first half of the P wave is larger than normal in lead V_1. When the right ventricular hypertrophy is due to obstructive lung disease and pulmonary emphysema the mean P vector may be directed at $+70°$ or more in the frontal plane (4).

There is an important exception to this rule. When the right ventricular hypertrophy is due to mitral stenosis, *left atrial abnormality* may still be present so a biatrial abnormality may be noted.

Direction of the Mean QRS Vector

When the systolic pressure overload of the right ventricle occurs after normal left ventricular preponderance has developed, the mean QRS vector shifts to a vertical position but may initially remain posteriorly directed. As time passes, the mean QRS vector becomes directed anteriorly.

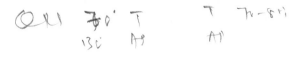

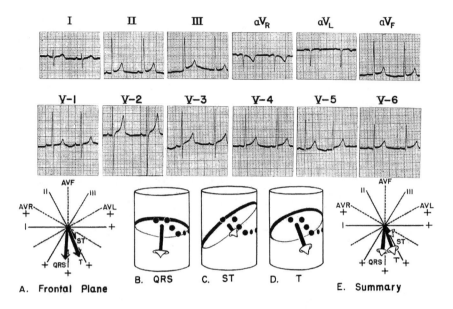

Figure 14-1 This electrocardiogram was recorded from an 8-year-old child with isolated pulmonary valve stenosis. The P waves are normal. The duration of the QRS complex is 0.07 second. In *A* and *B*, the large mean QRS vector is directed at +95° in the frontal plane and more than 10° anteriorly. It is directed toward the right ventricle. This is abnormal in an 8-year-old child; the mean QRS vector should be shifted more to the left and posteriorly at this age. In *A* and *D*, the mean T vector is directed at about +65° and about 30° anteriorly. In *C*, the S-T vector is directed almost parallel with the direction of the mean T vector; it is undoubtedly due also to repolarization forces. One would expect that the S-T and T vectors would be directed to the left and posteriorly. One hypothesis to explain the exception is that the transmyocardial pressure gradient in the right ventricle is presumably greater than normal, but the pressure in the endocardium is still greater than it is in the epicardial region. In addition, the normal repolarization of the left ventricle may now dominate the electrical field. (*Source*: Hurst JW, Woodson GC Jr. *Atlas of Spatial Vector Electrocardiography*. New York: The Blakiston Company, Inc, 1951:77. The author, J.W.H., owns the copyright.)

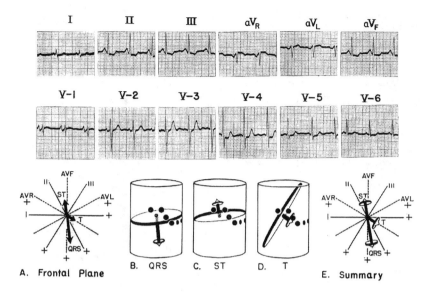

Figure 14-2 This electrocardiogram was recorded from a 35-year-old patient with mitral stenosis. The P waves are abnormal. The mean P vector is directed at about +80° in the frontal plane and an unknown amount anteriorly. Note that the P wave in lead II is almost 0.12 second in duration and more than two millimeters high. Note also that the amplitude of the first half of the P wave is two millimeters or more in lead V_1 and that the second half of the P wave measures about −0.045 millimeters/second. The second half of the P wave is negative in lead V_2. These abnormalities indicate both a left atrial abnormality and a right atrial abnormality. In A and B, the mean QRS vector is directed at about +80° in the frontal plane and about 30° posteriorly. In A and D, the small mean T vector is directed at +30° in the frontal plane and about 50° anteriorly, and in A and C, the mean S-T vector is directed at −95° in the frontal plane and about 10° anteriorly. The Q-T interval is 0.32 second. The vertical mean QRS vector that is still directed posteriorly is characteristic of systolic pressure overload such as occurs in adults with mitral stenosis. Later, the mean QRS vector will become more anteriorly directed. The left and right atrial abnormalities indicate that this patient was already developing pulmonary hypertension. The S-T and T wave vectors are characteristic of digitalis effect. (*Source:* Hurst JW, Woodson GC Jr. *Atlas of Spatial Vector Electrocardiography*. New York: The Blakiston Company, Inc, 1951:75. The author, J.W.H., owns the copyright.)

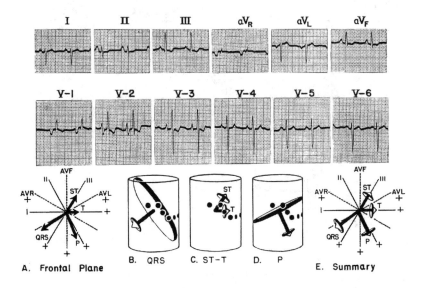

Figure 14-3 This electrocardiogram was recorded from a 38-year-old patient with mitral stenosis. The P waves are abnormal. In *A* and *D*, the mean vector for the P wave is directed about +70° in the frontal plane and 10° posteriorly. Note the notch at the midway point of the P wave in lead I, V_5 and V_6 and that the P wave is 2.5 mm high in lead II. The last half of the P wave is negative in leads V_1 and V_2. The area subtended by the last half of the P wave is −0.10 millimeters/second in size. There is a definite left atrial abnormality and possibly a slight right atrial abnormality. In *A* and *B*, the mean QRS vector is directed at about +145° in the frontal plane and about 20° to 30° anteriorly and the duration of the QRS complexes is 0.08 second. The QRS abnormality is typical of right ventricular hypertrophy. In *A* and *C*, the small mean T vector is directed at 0° in the frontal plane about 30° posteriorly, and the mean S-T vector is directed at about −60° in the frontal plane and about 30° posteriorly. The Q-T interval is 0.28 second. Left atrial abnormality plus right ventricular hypertrophy is commonly caused by mitral stenosis. This tracing illustrates the abnormalities that occur late in the natural history of mitral stenosis. The posteriorly directed small mean T vector is caused by right ventricular hypertrophy. The short Q-T interval and direction of the mean S-T vector in relationship to the mean T vector suggests digitalis effect. This electrocardiogram, showing

Amplitude of the QRS Complexes

The QRS complexes may be larger than normal, but there are no total QRS amplitude measurements that indicate right ventricular hypertrophy. Early in the course of the disease, the only sign of right ventricular hypertrophy may be an increase in the amplitude of the R wave in lead V_1; it may be 5 mm or greater. Also, if the amplitude of the R wave in lead V_1 is greater than the S wave, right ventricular hypertrophy may be present. These measurements, however, are considered to be minor signs of right ventricular hypertrophy. There is an important exception to the rule that the QRS amplitude increases when there is right ventricular hypertrophy; the right ventricular hypertrophy due to obstructive lung disease and emphysema may reveal low amplitude of the QRS complexes.

Direction of the Mean S-T and T Vectors

The mean S-T and T vectors may be directed to the left and posteriorly. The electrocardiograms shown in Figures 14-2 and 14-3 illustrate the electrocardiographic abnormalities of right ventricular hypertrophy due to mitral stenosis. The electrocardiographic abnormalities produced by obstructive lung disease and emphysema are discussed in Chapter 19.

---

advanced right ventricular hypertrophy, should be compared with the tracing shown in Figure 14.2. The tracing in Figure 14-2 shows a mean QRS vector that is directed vertically and posteriorly, representing an earlier stage of right ventricular hypertrophy due to mitral stenosis. (*Source*: Hurst JW, Woodson GC Jr. *Atlas of Spatial Vector Electrocardiography*. New York: The Blakiston Company, Inc, 1951:81. The author, J.W.H., owns the copyright.)

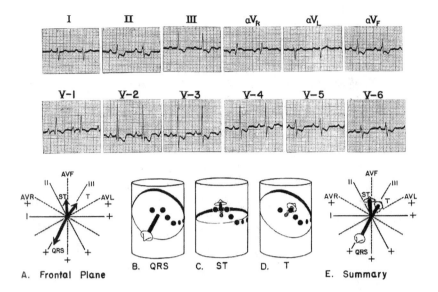

Figure 14-4 This electrocardiogram was recorded from a 38-year-old patient with an ostium secundum atrial septal defect. The P-R interval is 0.20 second and the duration of the QRS complex is 0.08 second. The mean P vector is directed at about +50° in the frontal plane and slightly anteriorly. The first half of the P wave is prominent in lead V_1, suggesting a right atrial abnormality. The second half of the P wave appears prominent but measures less than 0.03 millimeters/second. In A and B, the large mean QRS vector is directed at about +115° in the frontal plane and at least 80° anteriorly. Note that the largest portion of the QRS complex is produced by the middle and terminal portions of the deflections. This is in sharp contrast to the QRS complexes shown in Figure 14-1, where the initial 0.04 second of the QRS complex contributes the largest amount of ventricular QRS forces to the abnormality. The prominent terminal 0.02 to 0.03 forces in this tracing (14-4) are produced because there is a right ventricular conduction delay; the terminal 0.02 to 0.03 second vector is directed at about −170° in the frontal plane and parallel to the frontal plane. The mean T vector is directed about −60° in the frontal plane and at least 70° to 80° posteriorly. The mean S-T vector is directed at about −90° in the frontal plane and about 10° posteriorly. The Q-T interval is about 0.28 second. These abnormalities are caused by right ventricular hypertrophy and digi-

RIGHT VENTRICULAR HYPERTROPHY DUE TO DIASTOLIC PRESSURE OVERLOAD OF THE RIGHT VENTRICLE

There is only one common cause of isolated diastolic pressure overload of the right ventricle in adults: the ostium secundum atrial septal defect produces a large dilated right ventricle. Even in these patients, when the left-to-right shunt is great, there may be an associated increase in systolic pressure in the pulmonary artery and in the right ventricle causing some degree of systolic pressure overload of the right ventricle. There are rare causes of pure right ventricular diastolic pressure overload in adults, such as tricuspid valve regurgitation due to endocarditis, carcinoid heart disease, or myxomatous disease of the tricuspid valve. Also, there are rare causes of pulmonary valve regurgitation, such as congenital valve disease and endocarditis involving the pulmonary valve.

Diastolic pressure overload of the right ventricle should theoretically produce a mean QRS vector that is directed to the right and anteriorly and mean T and S-T vectors that are large and directed relatively parallel with the mean QRS vector. Such is not observed because a secundum atrial septal defect, the common cause of diastolic overload of the right ventricle, is always associated with a right ventricular conduction defect that prevents, or masks, the development of the theoret-

---

talis effect. The right atrial abnormality, the direction and size of the middle and terminal QRS vectors, and the direction of the S-T and T waves indicate right ventricular hypertrophy and right ventricular conduction delay that is often seen in patients with diastolic overload of the right ventricle, which is commonly due to ostium secundum atrial septal defect. The effect of digitalis is also noted. The right ventricular conduction delay masks the development of the expected features of pure diastolic overload of the right ventricle (see text). (*Source*: Hurst JW, Woodson GC Jr. *Atlas of Spatial Vector Electrocardiography*. New York: The Blakiston Company, Inc, 1951: 79. The author, J.W.H., owns the copyright.)

ical electrocardiographic features of diastolic pressure over-load of the right ventricle.

The electrocardiographic abnormalities that routinely oc-cur in patients with diastolic overload of the right ventricle due to an ostium secundum atrial septal defect are as follow:

Atrial fibrillation may be present.

The QRS duration may be normal, increased slightly, or sufficiently long to indicate right bundle branch block (QRS duration of 0.12 second).

The direction of the mean QRS vector is to the right and anteriorly, largely because a vector representing the *terminal portion* of the QRS complex is directed to the right and anteriorly, indicating a right ventricu-lar conduction delay. When the duration of the QRS complex is normal, this is referred to as right ventric-ular conduction delay.

The mean T and S-T vectors are usually directed to the left and posteriorly away from the right ventricle.

The electrocardiogram shown in Figure 14-4 illustrates the electrocardiographic abnormalities associated with a se-cundum atrial septal defect.

As described earlier, patients with ostium secundum atrial septal defect may develop Eisenmenger syndrome due to pulmonary arteriolar disease; this produces systolic pres-sure overload of the right ventricle.

REFERENCES

1. Cabrera E, Monroy JR. Systolic and diastolic loading of the heart. I. Physiologic and clinical data. Am Heart J 1952;43:661.

2. Cabrera E, Monroy JR. Systolic and diastolic loading of the heart. II. Electrocardiographic data. Am Heart J 1952;43:669.

3. Hurst JW. *Ventricular Electrocardiography*. New York: Gower Publishing, 1991;9:2.

4. Baljepally R, Spodick DH. Electrocardiographic screening for emphysema: The frontal plane P axis. Clin Cardiol 1999;22:226–228.

MYOCARDIAL INFARCTION CAN PRODUCE THE FOLLOWING ELECTROCARDIOGRAPHIC ABNORMALITIES (3)

The Dead Zone

The *dead zone* of most myocardial infarctions is usually located in the endocardial area of the left ventricle and occasionally in the endocardial area of the right ventricle (see Fig. 15-1). The dead zone is larger at the endocardium than it is at the epicardium. The dead area does not produce electrical forces. Accordingly, the electrical forces that are produced by the intact diametrically opposite ventricular myocardium dominate the electrical field and account for the abnormal Q waves that commonly occur with myocardial infarct. The direction of the vector representing the initial QRS forces is determined by the sum of the vectors produced by the depolarization of the normal endocardium plus those produced by the unbalanced depolarization forces that are produced opposite to the dead area. Therefore, a vector representing the initial 0.02 to 0.04 sec of the QRS complex tends to be directed away from the dead zone of infarction as shown in Figure 15-1A. This abnor-

---

Figure 15-1   The usual electrocardiographic signs of myocardial infarction. *A.* The "dead zone" of myocardial infarction is usually located in a segment of the left ventricle and occasionally in the right ventricle. The dead area is usually largest in the endocardium and smallest in the epicardium. The mean initial 0.03 to 0.04 QRS second vector is directed away from the "dead zone." *B.* The "dead zone" is surrounded by an area of "injury" that is larger at the epicardium than it is at the endocardium. The mean S-T vector produced by myocardial infarction is directed toward the area of predominant epicardial "injury." *C.* The area of "injury" is surrounded by an area of epicardial ischemia that is larger at the epicardium than at the endocardium. The mean T vector is commonly directed away from the area of predominant epicardial ischemia. Early in the course of infarction, the mean T vector may be directed toward the area of endocardial ischemia (see text).

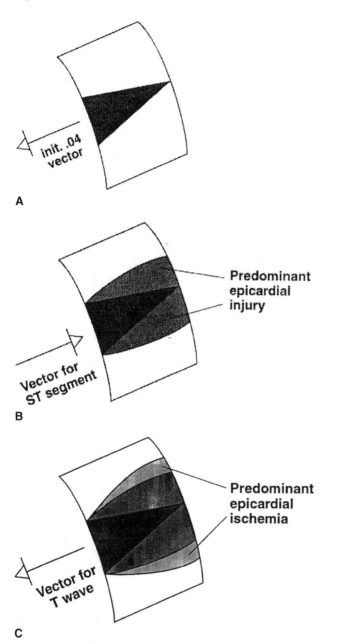

mality usually persists, but may gradually decrease in size or disappear.

The dead zone may occur in the mid portion of the myocardium or even in the epicardial area. In such cases the initial portion of the QRS complex will not be altered.

Segmental Epicardial Injury

The dead zone of the usual infarct is surrounded by an area of segmental predominant epicardial injury; the injured area is larger at the epicardium than it is at the endocardium. This creates an abnormal ST segment vector that is *directed toward* the epicardial injury surrounding the infarction, as shown in Figure 15-1B and Figure 15-2B. The S-T segment displacement decreases in amplitude as the hours and days pass. When the S-T segment displacement persists for weeks or months it is often caused by a ventricular aneurysm.

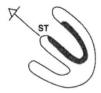

A. Generalized endocardial   B. Segmental epicardial   C. Generalized epicardial
          injury   injury   injury

Figure 15-2 The direction of the mean S-T vector caused by myocardial injury. *A*. The mean S-T segment vector is directed away from *generalized* endocardial injury as occurs with intense myocardial ischemia or infarction. *B*. The mean S-T vector is directed toward an area of *segmental* epicardial injury as occurs with the usual myocardial infarction. *C*. The mean S-T vector is directed toward the centroid of *generalized* epicardial injury due to myocardial ischemia or pericarditis. An exception to this rule occurs when there is an apical infarct, because the mean S-T vector may be directed toward a localized segment of the left ventricle which, being located at the cardiac apex, imitates generalized epicardial injury.

The genesis of the S-T segment displacement due to epicardial injury produced by myocardial infarction was described by Holland and Brooks (4,5). One theory holds that the electrical forces that create the S-T segment displacement are actually produced during the T-Q interval and that they are directed away from the area of epicardial injury. To accept this theory, one must believe that the depolarization process eliminates all electrical charges from the heart so that no electrical activity is possible until repolarization of the ventricles occurs. So, during the T-Q period the injured tissue creates its own electrical forces. The electrocardiographic machine senses the T-Q displacement and reacts by introducing an equal and opposite current to restore the normal baseline. Then, after the depolarization process removes all the electrical charges, the machine-induced artifact becomes apparent during the S-T segment. This produces a mean S-T segment vector that is directed toward the epicardial injury.

Some experts believe that the depolarization process does not remove all of the electrical charges from the ventricles. Accordingly, the vector representing the electrical forces are directed toward the injured epicardial tissue.

A third view of this interesting problem holds that both of the mechanisms are operative.

An abnormal S-T segment vector is usually a "pure" vector because in most patients, the pre-infarct normal tracing reveals no S-T segment displacement. Accordingly, unlike the new Q wave abnormality, or new T wave abnormality which are due to a combination of old normal electrical forces plus new abnormal electrical forces, the S-T vector is "pure."

Generalized Endocardial Injury

Endocardial injury produces an ST vector that is *directed away* from the centroid of generalized endocardial injury (see Fig. 15-2A). When the abnormality persists for several hours, a subendocardial infarct is likely. It is important to remember that subendocardial injury is usually generalized.

Generalized Epicardial Injury

Generalized epicardial injury may occur and this is discussed later in this chapter (see Figure 15-2C).

Segmental Epicardial Ischemia

The area of predominant epicardial injury of the usual infarct is surrounded by an area of segmental predominant epicardial ischemia; the ischemic area is larger at the epicardium than

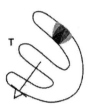

A. Segmental epicardial ischemia

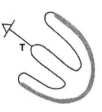

B. Generalized epicardial ischemia

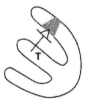

C. Segmental endocardial ischemia

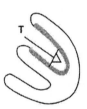

D. Generalized endocardial ischemia

Figure 15-3   The direction of the mean T vector produced by myocardial ischemia. *A.* The mean T vector may be directed away from *segmental* epicardial ischemia of the usual infarct. *B.* A large mean T vector may be directed away from the centroid of *generalized* epicardial ischemia such as occurs with cerebral catastrophies or hypertrophic cardiomyopathy. *C.* The mean T vector may be directed toward a *segment* of localized endocardial ischemia. This produces the hyperacute T waves of early infarction. *D.* The mean T vector may be directed toward the centroid of *generalized* endocardial ischemia. This occurs occasionally with infarction.

it is in the endocardium. This causes the mean T vector to be *directed away* from the area of predominant epicardial ischemia as shown in Figure 15–1C and Figure 15–3A. The T wave abnormality may gradually decrease in size and occasionally disappears.

Generalized epicardial ischemia may develop and this is discussed later in this chapter (see Figure 15-3B).

Epicardial myocardial ischemia delays the repolarization process in the region of the heart that is ischemic. This reverses the direction of the repolarization process in that area of the heart, causing the repolarization process to be directed predominately from endocardium to epicardium, producing an electrical force that is directed in the opposite direction. The direction of the vector representing the T waves is determined by the sum of vectors produced by the repolarization of the normal myocardium plus those produced by the altered repolarization in the ischemic myocardium.

Endocardial Ischemia

Endocardial ischemia may be segmental or generalized. This produces a large T vector that will be directed *toward a segment* of ischemic endocardium or *toward the centroid* of generalized endocardial ischemia (see Fig. 15-3C,D).

THE FOLLOWING POINTS DESERVE EMPHASIS

Epicardial dead zones will not produce abnormal Q waves and small intramural infarcts may not produce electrocardiographic abnormalities.

Infarcts may produce only one or two of the abnormalities discussed above. A non Q wave infarction in which S-T and T wave abnormalities occur, or only T wave abnormalities occur, is the classic example of this situation.

The direction of the mean S-T vector more accurately indicates the location of the infarction than does the direction of the mean Q and mean T vectors. Accordingly, the direction of the mean S-T vector should be used to identify the culprit coronary artery responsible for the infarction. This is true because the S-T segment vector is usually a new vector, whereas the initial Q wave abnormality of an infarct is the vector sum of the preexisting Q wave vector and the new Q wave abnormality due to infarction and the T wave abnormality of an infarct is the vector sum of the preexisting T wave vector plus the vector created by the new T wave abnormality of infarction.

The more infarcts a patient has, the less likely it is that the last infarct will reveal the expected abnormalities. This is true because the production of abnormal Q waves depends on an intact myocardial wall that is opposite to the new infarct. An old infarct that is located in the myocardium opposite to the new infarct eliminates the conditions needed to create a new Q wave vector. Also, the aortic and mitral valves are located opposite the left ventricular apex, so that a new abnormal Q wave may not be produced by an infarct located in that region of the left ventricle.

All of the abnormalities of infarction may disappear with the passage of time.

There are many electrocardiographic abnormalities that simulate myocardial infarction. These imitators in the electrocardiogram are referred to as pseudoinfarction and must be appreciated, else serious clinical errors will be made.

A MODEL TO STUDY

It is useful to use a Styrofoam cup and another half cup as a self-teaching aid (see Fig. 15-4). Place the whole cup in the anatomic position of the left ventricle and the half cup in the position of the right ventricle. Assume the origin of electrical activity is located in the center of the two cups and imagine that the hexaxial reference system of leads axes and the precordial lead axes are superimposed on the cups. It is useful to place a dead zone, with its accompanying areas of injury and

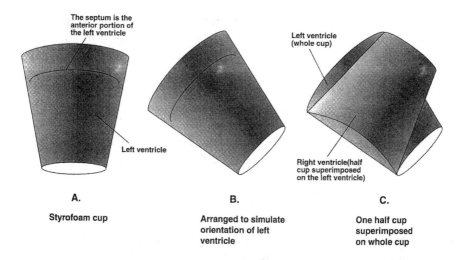

A.

Styrofoam cup

B.

Arranged to simulate
orientation of left
ventricle

C.

One half cup
superimposed
on whole cup

Figure 15-4 A teaching aid for visualizing the "projection" of the electrical forces associated with infarction on the 12 leads of the electrocardiogram. *A.* A Styrofoam cup simulates the left ventricle. *B.* The whole cup is turned counter clockwise and slightly anteriorly to simulate the exact location of the left ventricle and septum in the chest. *C.* One-half of a cup superimposed on a whole cup. The half cup simulates the right ventricle. Place the infarct anywhere within the left ventricle that you wish. Remember the initial mean 0.03 to 0.04 QRS vector is directed away from the endocardial dead zone, the mean S-T vector is directed toward epicardial injury, and the mean T vector is directed away from epicardial ischemia. Superimpose the hexaxial reference system and precordial lead axes onto the model and visualize how the three diagnostic vectors project onto the axes of the 12 leads. Once this task is performed with moderate speed, one should be able to survey a tracing and compute the direction of the diagnostic cardiac vectors, identify the presence of an infarct, determine the location of the infarct, and, at times, identify the culprit coronary artery.

ischemia, in different spots within the left ventricle (the whole cup) and predict the shape of the electrocardiographic deflections that would be recorded in the 12 leads. I have often used this test to determine if trainees really understood the vector concept or if they are memorizing vector positions rather than understanding how to use the concept. Accordingly, I suggest to the readers of this book that if this test cannot be completed, it would be useful to review the previous chapters and make certain the *six memories* are intact.

INFERIOR MYOCARDIAL INFARCTION

Inferior myocardial infarctions are usually caused by the abrupt occlusion of the mid or distal portion of the right coronary artery. Inferior myocardial infarction may also be caused by an acute obstruction of the branches of the circumflex coronary artery. And, though unusual, inferior myocardial infarction may be caused by the sudden occlusion of the left anterior descending coronary artery that wraps around the inferior surface of the left ventricle (6).

The usual inferior myocardial infarction produces the following abnormalities:

Sinus bradycardia may be present.

Atrioventricular block may be present.

A vector representing the initial 0.03 to 0.04 second of the QRS complex will be directed away from the inferior portion of the left ventricle. It is commonly directed at $-30°$ to $-60°$ in the frontal plane and slightly anterior. The initial 0.04 QRS vector will usually be directed superior to a horizontal mean QRS vector.

The mean ST vector, which is produced by predominant epicardial injury, will be directed toward the inferior surface of the left ventricle. It will usually be directed at $+90°$ to $+120°$ in the frontal plane and will be directed parallel to the frontal plane or slightly posterior.

The mean T vector, which is produced by predominant epicardial ischemia, will eventually be directed away from the inferior surface of the left ventricle. Early in the process of infarction, a hyperacute T wave vector may be directed toward the inferior segment of the left ventricle.

An electrocardiogram showing an acute inferior myocardial infarction is shown in Figure 15-5.

RIGHT VENTRICULAR MYOCARDIAL INFARCTION ASSOCIATED WITH INFERIOR MYOCARDIAL INFARCTION

Right ventricular infarction is almost always associated with an inferior myocardial infarction. It is commonly caused by the abrupt occlusion of the proximal portion of the right coronary artery prior to the first right ventricular branch (see Fig. 6-2).

Right ventricular infarction associated with an inferior myocardial infarction produces the following abnormalities:

The Q wave and T wave abnormalities that are commonly associated with inferior myocardial infarction are usually present.

The mean S-T vector, produced by epicardial injury, tends to be directed to the right and anteriorly toward the right ventricle. As a general rule, it will be directed between $+120°$ and $\pm180°$ in the frontal plane and varying degrees anteriorly. This produces S-T segment elevation in leads V_1 and V_2 and occasionally in leads V_3 and V_4. These findings may mislead the observer who has no knowledge of vector concepts into believing the patient has had an anterior myocardial in-

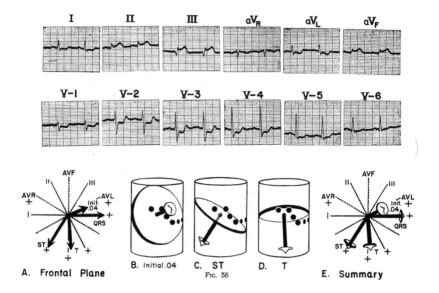

B. Initial .04   C. ST
A. Frontal Plane   Fɪɢ. 56   D. T   E. Summary

Figure 15-5 The electrocardiogram of a 62-year-old man showing inferior myocardial infarction. The P waves are normal and the duration of the P-R interval is 0.20 second. The duration of the QRS complex is about 0.08 second. The initial 0.04 QRS vector is directed at about $-25°$ in the frontal plane about $60°$ anteriorly. This suggests that the "dead zone" is located a little posteriorly as well as inferiorly. The mean S-T vector is directed at $+120°$ in the frontal plane and about $+20°$ to $+30°$ posteriorly. The direction of the S-T vector also suggests that the epicardial damage is located inferiorly and posteriorly. The mean T vector is directed inferiorly at about $+80°$ to $+90°$ in the frontal plane and more than $20°$ anteriorly. This abnormality is due to localized endocardial ischemia. The infarct is only 3 hours old and this type of hyperacute T wave abnormality can be seen at this time. Later, the mean T vector would undoubtedly be directed away from the evolving predominant epicardial ischemia. (*Source*: Hurst JW, Woodson GC Jr. *Atlas of Spatial Vector Electrocardiography*. New York: The Blakiston Division, Inc, 1952:125. The author, J.W.H., owns the copyright.)

farction. The true nature of the abnormality is recognized when it is noted that the mean S-T vector is directed to the *right* in the frontal plane as well as *anteriorly* where the right ventricle is located.

If an interpreter becomes fluent in determining the spatial direction of the mean S-T vector as described in this book, it is not necessary to record the deflection leads V_3R or V_4R as is often recommended by those who memorize patterns. Such extra precordial leads are not needed because it is quite easy to predict the deflections these extra leads will reveal.

Errors will be made if one simply memorizes that elevated S-T segments in leads V_3R and V_4R always indicates right ventricular infarction. For example, infarction of the septum may, at times, produce a mean S-T vector that is directed between $-90°$ and $\pm180°$ in the frontal plane and varying degrees anteriorly. The S-T segments may be elevated in leads V_3R and V_4R in such patients, suggesting right ventricular infarction. Also, the S-T segment vector due to subendocardial infarction may be directed between $-90°$ and $\pm180°$ in the frontal plane and varying degrees anteriorly. This may produce S-T segment elevation in leads V_3R and V_4R suggesting right ventricular infarction. The frontal plane direction of the mean S-T segment vector is usually directed to the *left* in the frontal plane and *anteriorly* when there is an anterior or anterolateral myocardial infarction. In rare cases the S-T segments may be elevated in leads V, R and V_4R in these patients. The establishment of the spatial direction of the mean S-T segment vector usually identifies the correct location of the infarction.

To repeat for emphasis, the person who memorizes patterns usually disassociates the frontal plane direction of electrical forces from the anteroposterior direction of the same electrical forces and is likely to misinterpret the deflections recorded in the right-sided precordial leads as being due to right ventricular infarction.

An electrocardiogram showing right ventricular infarction associated with inferior infarction is shown in Figure 15-6.

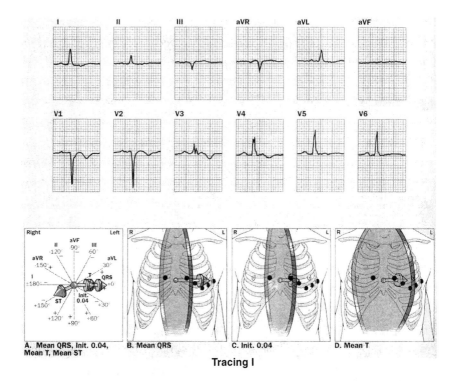

Tracing I

Figure 15-6 Electrocardiograms showing the development of an inferior and right ventricular infarction. These electrocardiograms, showing the development of a right ventricular infarction, were recorded from a 51-year-old man. He had an anterior infarction in August 1988. A coronary arteriogram made at that time revealed total obstruction of the first diagonal coronary artery and the left anterior descending coronary artery after the first septal perforator. The patient had coronary bypass surgery the same month. He developed recurrent ventricular tachycardia that could not be controlled with drugs, including amiodarone. Electrophysiologic testing with endocardial mapping and possible endocardial surgical resection was planned. It seemed wise to perform a coronary arteriogram prior to these procedures in order to determine whether myocardial ischemia might be responsible for the patient's arrhythmia.

The arteriogram was made on November 29, 1988. Unfortunately, the procedure precipitated severe dissection of the right coronary artery, which became completely occluded. The patient was

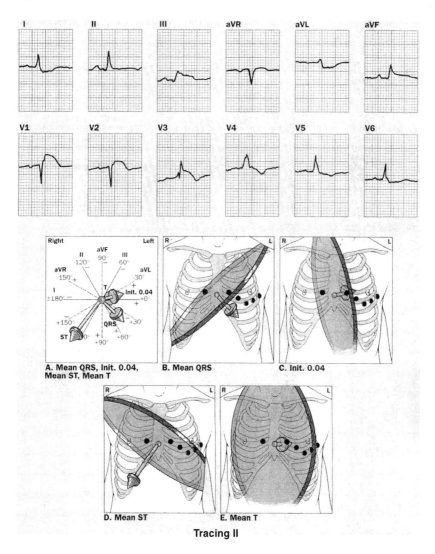

A. Mean QRS, Init. 0.04, Mean ST, Mean T

B. Mean QRS

C. Init. 0.04

D. Mean ST

E. Mean T

Tracing II

Figure 15-6 Continued
transferred to Emory University Hospital, where percutaneous
transluminal coronary angioplasty was unsuccessful; the proximal
portion of the right coronary artery became completely obstructed.
These events made it possible to study the evolution of a right ventricular myocardial infarction occurring in the presence of a former
anteroseptal myocardial infarction. The patient responded to the
specific treatment for right ventricular infarction.

Tracing I. This electrocardiogram was recorded at 7:24 p.m. on
November 29, 1988, after coronary arteriography, at which time a
severe dissection of the right coronary artery occurred. It shows the
previous anteroseptal infarction due to total occlusion of the left anterior descending artery.

The rhythm is normal; there are 72 complexes per minute. The
duration of the PR interval is 0.17 second. The duration of the QRS
complex is 0.09 second and that of the QT interval is 0.37 second. *P
waves*: The P waves are normal. *QRS complex*: The mean QRS vector
is directed at 0° in the frontal plane. It is directed at about 20° to
30° posteriorly, and the mean initial 0.04 second vector is directed
about 20° posteriorly—a little more than it should be for this particular mean QRS vector. *T waves*: The mean T vector is directed at
0° in the frontal plane, and 80° posteriorly, away from an area of
anterior epicardial ischemia. *A.* The frontal plane projections of the
mean QRS, mean initial 0.04 second QRS, mean ST segment, and
mean T vectors. *B–D.* The spatial orientations of the mean QRS,
mean initial 0.04 second QRS, and mean T vectors, are shown respectively.

Tracing II. This electrocardiogram was recorded at 11:46 p.m.,
after an attempted angioplasty to open the totally occluded right
coronary artery. A more proximal portion of this vessel became completely obstructed, at which time the electrocardiogram showed evidence of right ventricular infarction. The rhythm is normal. There
are 80 complexes per minute. The duration of the PR interval is 0.20
second. The duration of the QRS complex is 0.10 second, and the
duration of the QT interval is 0.36 second. *P waves*: The P waves
are normal, although the mean P vector is a little more posteriorly
directed than in the tracing shown in Figure 15.6(1). *QRS complex*:
The mean QRS vector is directed +45° inferiorly, and 15° posteriorly. The mean initial 0.04 second QRS vector is directed a little
more to the left than it was in Figure 15.6(I); this may be due to a

new inferior dead zone. *ST segment*: The mean ST vector is huge. It is directed about $+130°$ to the right, and $40°$ to $60°$ anteriorly. This is characteristic of epicardial injury associated with inferior and right ventricular infarction. Note the epsilon waves in the S-T segment in leads V_1 and V_2. *T waves*: The mean T vector is directed markedly posteriorly. It is difficult to identify the frontal plane projection of the mean T vector, but the T waves are definitely inverted in lead V_1 through V_5. The vector is directed away from an area of anterior epicardial ischemia. *A*. This figure shows the frontal plane projections of the mean QRS, mean initial 0.04 second QRS, mean ST, and mean T vectors. *B–E*. The spatial orientations of the mean QRS, mean initial 0.04 second QRS, mean ST, and mean T vectors, are shown respectively.

Summary: Tracing I shows an anteroseptal infarction. The unusual electrocardiogram shown in part II exhibits abnormalities characteristic of right ventricular infarction. Tracing II followed coronary angioplasty, which was performed to open the right coronary artery, which was completely occluded due to dissection associated with arteriography. The mean S-T segment vector is directed to the right and anteriorly in tracing II. A tracing made from electrode position V_3R would undoubtedly show an elevated ST segment. The direction of the mean ST segment vector is a better indicator of the culprit artery than that of the mean initial 0.04 second QRS or the mean T vector. (*Source*: Hurst JW. *Ventricular Electrocardiography*. New York: Gower Medical Publishing, 1991:11.18, 11.19. The author, J.W.H., owns the copyright.)

TRUE POSTERIOR MYOCARDIAL INFARCTION

A true posterior myocardial infarction is usually caused by the abrupt occlusion of posterior marginal branches of the circumflex coronary artery. It produces the following abnormalities:

The initial 0.03 to 0.04 second QRS vector is directed anteriorly away from the endocardial dead zone located in a true posterior segment of the left ventricle. This

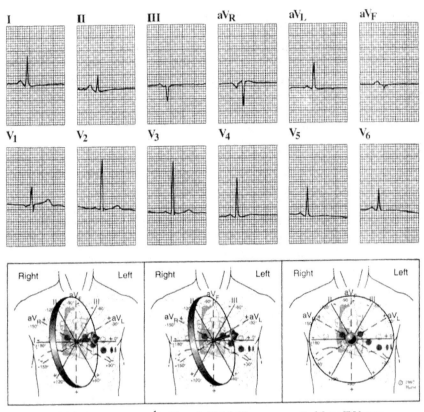

a. Mean QRS Vector   b. Mean Initial 0.04   c. Mean T Vector
                            Second Vector

Figure 15-7 This electrocardiogram was recorded from a man with a true posterior infarcton. The P waves are normal and the P-R interval is 0.15 to 0.16 second. The duration of the QRS complex is 0.07 to 0.08 second. The mean QRS vector and the mean initial 0.04 QRS vector are directed at $-10°$ in the frontal plane and at least $45°$ anteriorly. The mean T vector is directed about $90°$ anteriorly. There are four possible causes of these abnormalities. Right ventricular hypertrophy could produce the anterior direction of the mean QRS vector and the mean initial 0.04 QRS vector, but it would be most unusual for the frontal plane direction of the mean QRS vector to be at $-10°$. In addition the mean T vector would be directed to the left and posteriorly, whereas in this tracing it is directed anteriorly. Preexcitation produces a large R wave in leads V_1 and V_2. The mean QRS vector is usually directed normally when viewed in the frontal plane.

The mean S-T vector is directed posteriorly, toward the predominant epicardial injury surrounding the true posterior dead zone.

The mean T vector is directed anteriorly, away from the predominant epicardial ischemia surrounding the true posterior infarction.

The tall R waves in leads V_1 and V_2 must be differentiated from a similar finding caused by right ventricular hypertrophy. As a rule, the mean QRS vector will be directed vertically or to the right and anteriorly in patients with right ventricular hypertrophy, whereas the frontal plane direction of the mean QRS vector is directed normally in patients with a true posterior myocardial infarction.

The initial 0.03 to 0.04 sec QRS vector may be directed anteriorly in patients with Duchenne muscular dystrophy with associated cardiomyopathy. This abnormality is caused

---

of the ventricles could cause the mean QRS vector to be directed anteriorly, but in this tracing there is no delta wave. The cardiomyopathy associated with Duchenne muscular dystrophy can produce a QRS vector to be directed anteriorly because of the myocardial fibrosis located predominantly in the posterior portion of the left ventricle. Finally, a true posterior infarction is the most likely cause of the abnormal mean QRS vector, 0.04 QRS vector, and mean T vector. A coronary arteriogram revealed 40% obstruction of the left main coronary artery, 60% to 70% obstruction of a ramus artery, 70% to 80% obstruction of an obtuse marginal artery, 50% obstruction of the ostium of the right coronary artery, and 90% obstruction of the proximal portion of the right coronary artery. (*Source*: Hurst JW. *Cardiovascular Diagnosis. The Initial Examination*. St. Louis: Mosby-Year Book, Inc, 1993:374. The author, J.W.H., owns the copyright.)

by an area of endocardial fibrosis in the posterior portion of
the left ventricle in patients with this disease (7).

The initial 0.03–.04 sec QRS vector may be directed anteriorly in patients with pre-excitation of the ventricles. The
delta wave and prolonged QRS duration allow the interpreter
to identify this abnormality.

An electrocardiogram showing a true posterior infarction
is shown in Figure 15-7.

SEPTAL AND ANTEROSEPTAL INFARCTION

The interventricular septum is the anterior portion of the left
ventricle (see Fig. 6-1C,D). Because of its unique position, a
myocardial infarction located in that area of the myocardium
may be localized to the septum, or more commonly extend to
the anterior portion of the left ventricle.

A septal infarct may be caused by the sudden obstruction
of the septal branch of the left anterior descending coronary
artery and a large anteroseptal infarction may be caused by
the sudden obstruction of the left anterior descending coronary artery or its branches.

Myocardial infarcts commonly produce abnormal Q
waves in the electrocardiogram. Such abnormal Q waves are
produced by the removal of electrical forces in the region of
the infarct, which permits the electrical forces produced by the
opposite wall to dominate the electrical field during the first
0.03 to 0.04 second of the QRS complex. However, the abnormal initial QRS forces produced by septal infarction may be
no more than 0.02 second in duration. This is true because
normal septal depolarization occurs during the first 0.01 to
0.02 second of the QRS. These forces are removed when there
is septal infarction. Accordingly, the R waves in leads V_1, V_2,
and even V_3 may be eliminated. Such isolated poor "R wave
progression" should not be labeled as a definite septal infarction, because there are other causes of the abnormality.

For instance, left ventricular hypertrophy due to systolic pressure overload of the left ventricle may occasionally produce "poor R wave progression" in the precordial leads. When the initial 0.01 or 0.02 second QRS vector is posterior to the subsequent QRS vectors, septal infarct is usually the cause. This produces no R wave in leads V_1 and V_2 and a Q wave followed by an R wave and S wave in lead V_3; these abnormalities are greatly different from "the absent R wave progression" rubric. This abnormality commonly occurs with septal infarct or anteroseptal infarction.

The mean S-T vector due to septal infarction is directed anteriorly. Theoretically, it can be directed in almost any direction in the frontal plane, depending on the exact location of the septum in a particular patient. For example, the mean S-T segment vector may be directed in the right upper quadrant ($-90°$ to $\pm180°$) of the hexaxial reference system when the first septal branch of the left anterior descending coronary artery is injected with alcohol for the induction of infarction in patients with idiopathic hypertrophic cardiomyopathy. When an S-T segment vector is directed in that direction, it could possibly imitate the S-T segment abnormalities of right ventricular infarction, including S-T segment elevations in leads V_3R and V_4R. There are, however, other signs of septal infarction, such as the Q wave abnormality described above, and no QRS signs of inferior infarction. The mean S-T segment vector of anteroseptal infarction is usually directed to the left and anteriorly. It could be directed inferiorly to the extent that an elevation of the S-T segment could be recorded in leads V_3R and V_4R, suggesting right ventricular infarction. There are, however, other signs of anteroseptal infarction, such as the Q waves described above, and no QRS signs of inferior infarction.

The direction of the mean S-T vector due to septal or anteroseptal myocardial infarction is obviously determined by the exact location of the infarct; the location of the interventricular septum itself, because a slight variance in its position may

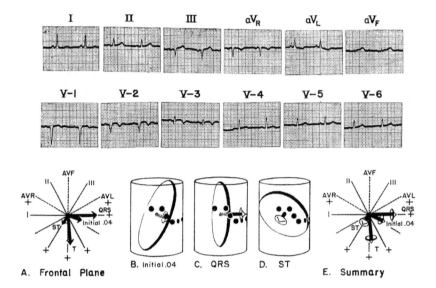

Figure 15-8 This electrocardiogram, recorded on a 62-year-old patient, shows an anteroseptal myocardial infarction. The P waves are normal and the P-R interval is 0.15 second. The duration of the QRS complex is 0.08 second. The direction of the mean QRS vector is about 0° in the frontal plane and about 15° posterior. The direction of the mean initial 0.04 second QRS vector is at about +25° to +30° in the frontal plane and about 25° posterior. Note that the initial 0.02 second QRS forces are posterior to the subsequent forces; this signifies the presence of septal involvement. This produces an absent R wave in leads V_1 and V_2 and a small Q wave followed by an R wave and S wave in lead V_3. The mean S-T vector is directed at +120° in the frontal plane and at least 45° anteriorly. The mean T vector is directed at +85° in the frontal plane and about 30° to 40° posterior. The U wave is abnormally large in leads V_1-V_3. The septal infarction can be recognized because the initial QRS forces are directed more posteriorly than the subsequent QRS forces. This abnormality produces absent initial R waves in leads V_1 and V_2, but produces a Q wave followed by an R wave in lead V_3. This is characteristic of septal infarction and is more diagnostic than an absent R wave in lead V_1–V_3, which can be caused by septal infarct but can also be caused by left ventricular hypertrophy due to systolic pressure overload of the left ventricle. The S-T segment vector is directed to the right and

alter the direction of the S-T vector considerably; and the thickness of the left ventricular myocardium, including the septum.

The mean T vector is usually directed to the left and posteriorly when it is related to a septal or anteroseptal infarction. It is usually located more to the left and more posteriorly when the anterior portion of the left ventricle is involved along with the septum, as compared to the direction of the mean T vector caused by an isolated infarction of the septum.

An electrocardiogram showing an anteroseptal infarction is shown in Figure 15-8.

ANTEROLATERAL MYOCARDIAL INFARCTION

Infarction of the anterolateral portion of the left ventricle is usually caused by abrupt occlusion of the left anterior descending coronary artery, or one of its diagonal branches. The occlusion may be in the first portion of the left anterior de-

---

anteriorly. This should always force an interpreter to consider the possibility of right ventricular infarction. As stated earlier, generalized endocardial injury as well as anteroseptal or septal infarction can cause the S-T segment vector to be directed to the right and anteriorly, suggesting right ventricular infarction. The current impression is that the S-T segment vector caused by right ventricular infarction is usually directed from about $+120°$ to $+180°$ whereas the S-T segment vectors of septal infarctions or subendocardial injury are usually directed between $-90°$ to $\pm180°$. In addition the S-T segment vector associated with right ventricular infarction usually occurs in patients with other electrocardiographic signs of inferior myocardial infarction. Note that the initial QRS forces in this tracing do not indicate the presence of an inferior infarction and do indicate the presence of a septal infarction. (*Source*: Hurst JW, Woodson GC Jr. *Atlas of Spatial Vector Electrocardiography*. New York: The Blakiston Division, Inc, 1952:149. The author, J.W.H., owns the copyright.)

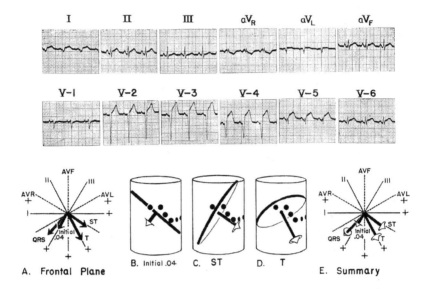

Figure 15-9 This electrocardiogram, showing anterolateral myocardial infarction, was recorded from a 59-year-old patient. The P waves are normal and the P-R interval is 0.12 second. The duration of the QRS complexes is 0.08 to 0.09 second. The mean QRS vector is directed at about +135° in the frontal plane and at least 70° posterior. The initial 0.04 second QRS vector is directed at about +120° in the frontal plane and is parallel with the frontal plane. The large mean S-T vector is directed at +30° in the frontal plane and about 10° anterior. The large mean T vector is directed at +50° to +60° in the frontal plane and about 10° to 20° anterior. The initial 0.04 second QRS vector is directed away from an anterolateral infarction. The mean S-T vector is directed toward the anterolateral epicardial injury. The mean hyperacute T wave vector is directed toward anterior-lateral endocardial ischemia. One should expect the S-T segment vector to gradually decrease in size and the mean T vector to be redirected away from the area of epicardial anterolateral ischemia. (*Source*: Hurst JW, Woodson GC Jr: *Atlas of Spatial Vector Electrocardiography*. New York: The Blakiston Division, Inc, 1952:143. The author, J.W.H., owns the copyright.)

scending artery or anywhere in the first one-third to one-half of that artery.

Anterolateral myocardial infarction produces the following electrocardiographic abnormalities:

> The initial 0.03 to 0.04 second QRS vector is directed to the right and posteriorly away from the anterolateral dead zone.
>
> The mean S-T vector is directed to the left and parallel with the frontal plane or anteriorly toward the area of predominant epicardial injury surrounding the infarction. Leads V_3R and V_4R could possibly show elevated S-T segments when the mean S-T vector is directed a little more inferiorly and anteriorly than usual. This could lead an interpreter who memorizes patterns to erroneously believe there is a right ventricular infarction.
>
> The mean T vector is directed to the right and posteriorly away from the area of predominant epicardial ischemia surrounding the infarction. Initially, of course, a large hyperacute mean T vector may be directed toward the area of segmental endocardial ischemia.

The electrocardiogram of anterolateral myocardial infarction is shown in Figure 15-9.

APICAL MYOCARDIAL INFARCTION

The rare infarction of the apex (or near the apex) of the left ventricle may be caused by the abrupt closure of a diagonal branch of the left anterior descending coronary artery. It can be caused by the abrupt occlusion of the obtuse margin of the circumflex coronary artery and rarely from occlusion of the distal branches of the right coronary artery. The patient may

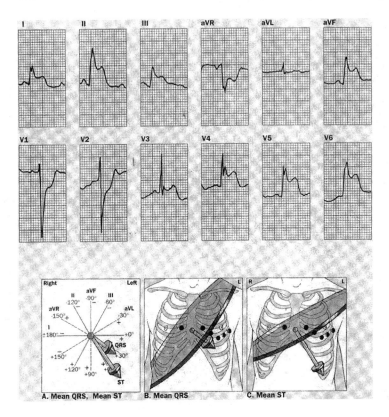

Figure 15-10 This electrocardiogram showing an apical myocardial infarction was recorded from a 52-year-old man. The P waves are normal and the P-R interval is 0.12 second. The duration of the QRS complexes is 0.10 second. The mean QRS vector is directed at +35° to +40° in the frontal plane and about 15° to 20° posterior. The initial 0.04 second QRS vector is directed at about +60° to +70° in the frontal plane and at least 20° anteriorly. The large mean S-T vector is directed at about +60° in the frontal plane and 15° to 20° posteriorly. The mean T vector is directed at about +50° in the frontal plane and about 20° anteriorly. The differential diagnosis is between apical infarction and pericarditis. As discussed in the chapter on pericarditis, the mean S-T vector is directed toward the centroid of generalized epicardial injury. The S-T vector of apical infarction is also directed toward the cardiac apex even though the epicardial injury is segmental. No abnormal Q waves are seen in

have triple-vessel atherosclerotic coronary heart disease and either one of the vessels just mentioned may be the culprit artery.

Apical myocardial infarction produces the following electrocardiographic abnormalities:

There may be no abnormal Q wave because there is no myocardial tissue opposite the cardiac apex; the aortic and mitral valves are located opposite the cardiac apex.

The mean S-T vector is directed toward the predominant epicardial injury located at the cardiac apex. This produces elevated S-T segments in leads I, II, III, aV_L, aV_F, and V_2–V_6. The direction of S-T segment vector is similar to that seen in generalized pericarditis.

The mean T vector tends to be directed away from the predominant epicardial ischemia located around the infarct. This produces a T vector that is directed away from the cardiac apex. This, too, is similar to the T wave abnormality caused by pericarditis.

---

either condition because the endocardium is intact in pericarditis and there is no myocardium opposite an apical infarct to generate an abnormal Q wave. It is not always possible to separate these two conditions. However, when the S-T segment displacement is extremely large, as it is in this patient, infarct is the likely diagnosis. The problem with this approach is that infarcts do not always create extremely large S-T segment displacement. A coronary arteriogram in this patient revealed 100 percent occlusion of the right coronary artery, 68 percent diameter obstruction of the circumflex coronary artery, 50 percent diameter obstruction of the first marginal coronary artery, and only 25 percent diameter obstruction of the left anterior descending coronary artery. (*Source*: Hurst JW. *Ventricular Electrocardiography*. New York: Gower Medical Publishing, 1991: 11. 26. The author, J.W.H., owns the copyright.)

It may be difficult to differentiate the electrocardio-graphic abnormalities caused by generalized pericarditis from the electrocardiographic abnormalities associated with apical (or near apical) myocardial infarction. Infarction is favored whenever the abnormal ST vector is huge and the abnormal T vector is small, but such abnormalities are not always present. Accordingly, other clinical data must be used to separate peri-carditis from apical infarction.

An electrocardiogram showing apical myocardial in-farction is shown in Figure 15-10.

NON–Q WAVE MYOCARDIAL INFARCTION

A non–Q wave infarction produces the following electrocardio-graphic abnormalities:

Abnormal Q waves are not always produced by myocar-dial infarction. Normally, the initial 0.02 to 0.04 por-tion of the QRS complex is produced by the depolar-ization of the septum and endocardium of both ventricles. A finite amount of infarcted myocardium must be damaged so that depolarization is not possi-ble in a portion of the endocardium of the left and, occasionally, the right ventricle in order for an ab-normal Q wave to be produced. Accordingly, small areas of infarction may not produce abnormal Q waves in the electrocardiogram. In addition, there must be viable myocardium opposite the dead zone due to infarction in order for an abnormal Q wave to be produced in the electrocardiogram. This is why new infarcts may not produce electrocardiographic abnormalities in a patient who has had previous in-farcts. It is also why abnormal Q waves do not de-velop in patients with apical infarcts; the aortic and mitral valves are opposite the apical dead area. Infarcts that are intramural or epicardial in location will not produce abnormal Q waves. Finally, abnormal Q waves may actually disappear with the passage of time.

The typical S-T segment and T wave abnormalities may be evident when there is a "non-Q wave" infarction. The mean ST segment vector is directed toward predominant epicardial injury, and the mean T vector is directed away from predominant epicardial ischemia.

The patient who has chest discomfort that is characteristic of prolonged myocardial ischemia and a rise in the serum cardiac enzymes with only S-T and T wave abnormalities, or only T wave abnormalities, is said to have a "non–Q wave" infarction.

Formerly, a "non–Q wave" infarct was referred to as a "non-transmural" infarction and an infarct showing abnormal Q waves was referred to as a "transmural" infarct. This designation is no longer used, because, when studied at autopsy, some transmural infarcts reveal no abnormal Q waves and some non-transmural infarcts reveal abnormal Q waves. In other words, the anatomic correlate is not justified.

An electrocardiogram of a non-Q wave infarction is shown in Figure 15-11.

ABNORMAL S-T SEGMENTS AS SIGNS OF MYOCARDIAL INJURY

Endocardial Injury

Generalized Endocardial Injury

Endocardial injury is usually generalized and produces a mean S-T vector that is directed opposite to the centroid of the left ventricular endocardium (see Fig. 15-2A). When the S-T segment vector persists for several hours, a generalized left

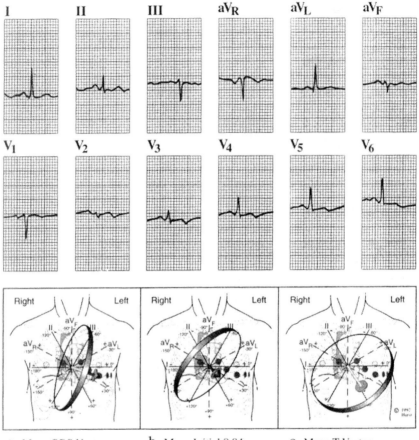

a. Mean QRS Vector   b. Mean Initial 0.04   c. Mean T Vector
                         Second Vector

Figure 15-11 This electrocardiogram, showing a non–Q wave infarction, was recorded from a 62-year-old man with unstable angina
pectoris who had several episodes of prolonged chest discomfort that
was characteristic of the pain produced by prolonged myocardial
ischemia. The P waves are normal and the P-R interval is 0.12 second. The duration of the QRS complexes is 0.08 second. The mean
QRS vector is directed at about +15° in the frontal plane and about
20° posteriorly. The initial 0.04 second QRS vector is directed at
about +40° in the frontal plane and 30° to 40° anteriorly. The mean

ventricular endocardial infarction can be identified. At autopsy the entire left ventricular endocardium may be infarcted.

A generalized left ventricular endocardial infarction is usually caused by one of the following pathophysiologic states. There may be severe triple-vessel coronary atherosclerotic disease with abrupt occlusion of one of the vessels (usually the left anterior descending coronary artery) or abrupt obstruction of the left main coronary artery. Also, the following conditions may be present. The patient may have left ventricular hypertrophy, elevated left ventricular diastolic pressure, moderate coronary atherosclerosis of several vessels, and hypotension due to any cause (such as gastrointestinal bleeding). In the latter case, the hypotension may decrease the coronary artery–left ventricular diastolic pressure gradient so that myocardial perfusion is profoundly reduced when hypotension develops, leading to generalized endocardial injury and infarction.

An electrocardiogram showing endocardial infarction is shown in Figure 15–12.

Epicardial Injury

Segmental Epicardial Injury

The mean S-T vector is directed toward the segmental predominant epicardial injury that occurs in the usual infarction (see Figs. 15-1B and 15-2B).

T vector is directed at about +55° in the frontal plane and 80° to 90° posterior. The T wave abnormality is the only definite abnormality seen in this tracing. The clinical history, plus the T wave abnormality, permits the diagnosis of non–Q wave infarction. (*Source*: Hurst JW. *Cardiovascular Diagnosis. The Initial Examination*. St. Louis: Mosby-Year Book, Inc, 1993:382. The author, J.W.H., owns the copyright.)

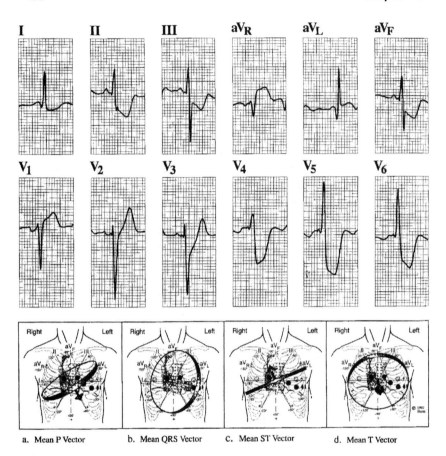

a. Mean P Vector   b. Mean QRS Vector   c. Mean ST Vector   d. Mean T Vector

Figure 15-12 This electrocardiogram, showing endocardial infarction, was recorded from a 54-year-old hypertensive man who had prolonged severe retrosternal pain. He developed ventricular fibrillation and was resuscitated successfully. There is left atrial abnormality and the P-R interval is 0.13 second. The duration of the QRS complex is 0.09 second. The mean QRS vector is directed at about +15° in the frontal plane and about 70° posteriorly. The mean S-T vector is huge. It is directed at about −115° in the frontal plane and is parallel with the frontal plane. The S-T vector is directed away from generalized endocardial injury. When this type of generalized endocardial injury persists, it signifies the presence of a generalized left ventricular endocardial infarction. Such patients usually have

Generalized Epicardial Injury

Generalized epicardial injury as illustrated in Figure 15-2C can be caused by pericarditis or can be imitated by apical infarction. (See discussion earlier under Apical Infarction.)

ABNORMAL T WAVES AS SIGNS OF MYOCARDIAL ISCHEMIA

There are four types of abnormal T waves that may signal an early stage of myocardial infarction. Endocardial myocardial ischemia may be segmental or generalized and epicardial myocardial ischemia may also be segmental or generalized.

Endocardial Ischemia

Segmental Endocardial Ischemia

Segmental endocardial ischemia can be recognized when the mean T vector becomes abruptly large and is directed toward an area of segmental endocardial ischemia. This is referred to as a *hyperacute T wave abnormality* (see Fig. 15-3C). An S-T segment vector accompanies the large T waves and is probably caused by large repolarization forces. The T waves may resemble the T waves associated with hyperkalemia, which are large and peaked. The large mean T vector may be directed about +30° to +60° inferiorly and anteriorly when there is an abrupt occlusion of the proximal portion of the left anterior descending coronary artery, and it may be directed about +90° to +120° inferiorly and parallel with the frontal plane when it

---

triple-vessel coronary atherosclerosis or obstruction of the left main coronary artery. This unique tracing is likely to appear when there is obstructive coronary atherosclerosis, left ventricular hypertrophy, elevated diastolic pressure in the left ventricle, and hypotension from any cause. (*Source*: Hurst JW. *Cardiac Puzzles*. St. Louis: Mosby-Year Book, Inc, 1995:77. Used with permission.)

is caused by an abrupt occlusion of the mid or distal portion of the right coronary artery (see Fig. 15-13).

Generalized Endocardial Ischemia

On rare occasions the vector representing the large *hyperacute T wave* abnormality may be directed toward the centroid of *generalized endocardial ischemia* (see Figs. 15-3D and 15-14).

Epicardial Ischemia

Segmental Epicardial Ischemia

The mean T vector is directed away from the *segment of epicardium* that is ischemic. This type of T wave abnormality occurs commonly with most infarcts (see Fig. 15-3A). Such an abnormality, appearing as the sole abnormality in the proper clinical setting, may be due to a "non–Q wave infarct" as shown in Figure 15–11.

Generalized Epicardial Ischemia

As shown in Figure 15-3B, this type of T wave abnormality may develop in patients with an acute cerebral vascular catastrophe such as subarachnoid hemorrhage. We now believe that these events can cause instantaneous stimulation of the sympathetic nervous system, which causes myocyte damage through the release of catecholamines at the cellular level, or can produce a catecholamine storm, similar to cocaine toxicity, that causes intense generalized epicardial coronary artery spasm (see Fig. 15-15). This type of T wave abnormality can also be due to a nonischemic cause. For example, pericarditis, which is usually generalized, may produce a nonischemic epicardial damage that alters the direction of the repolarization process. A similar T wave abnormality of this type may be chronically present in patients with apical hypertrophy cardiomyopathy.

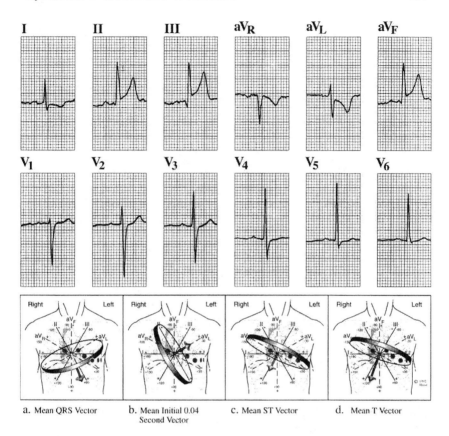

a. Mean QRS Vector   b. Mean Initial 0.04   c. Mean ST Vector   d. Mean T Vector
                         Second Vector

Figure 15-13   This electrocardiogram, showing *segmental inferior endocardial ischemia*, was recorded from a 44-year-old man with an acute inferior infarction. The purpose in showing this figure is to emphasize that *hyperacute T waves* may be the first sign of impending myocardial infarction. (*Source*: Hurst JW. *Cardiovascular Diagnosis. The Initial Examination*. St. Louis: Mosby-Year Book, Inc, 1993:368. The author, J.W.H., owns the copyright.)

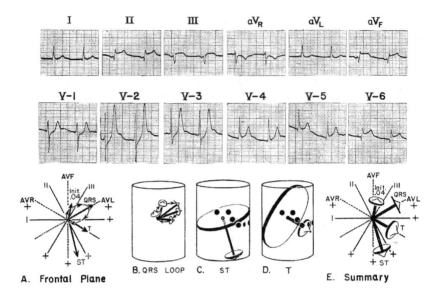

Figure 15-14 This electrocardiogram, showing an acute inferior-lateral myocardial infarction and *generalized endocardial ischemia*, was recorded from a 55-year-old patient. Note in A and B the initial 0.04 second QRS vector is directed superiorly and anteriorly, producing an abnormal Q wave in II, III, aV$_F$ and a large R wave in leads V$_1$ and V$_2$. The mean S-T vector is directed at +75° in the frontal plane and about 30° posteriorly, indicating inferior-posterior epicardial injury. The hyperacute mean T vector is huge and is directed at +30° in the frontal plane and at least 30° anteriorly, signifying *severe generalized endocardial ischemia*. (Source: Hurst JW, Woodson GC Jr. *Atlas of Spatial Vector Electrocardiography*. New York: The Blakiston Company, Inc, 1951:123. The author, J.W.H., owns the copyright.)

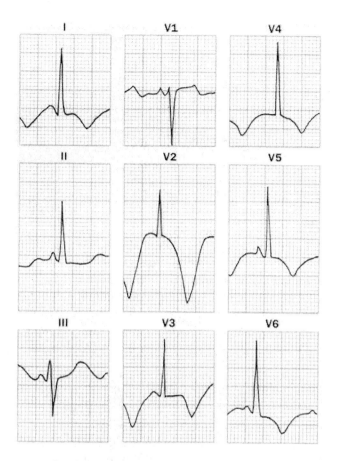

Figure 15-15 This electrocardiogram, showing *generalized epicardial ischemia*, was recorded from a patient with subarachnoid hemorrhage. Note the large "Niagara Falls" T waves. The huge mean T vector is directed at about +135° in the frontal plane and is parallel with the frontal plane. Such cerebral T waves may occur with any acute cerebral catastrophe. We now believe that this type of abnormality is the result of intense generalized epicardial ischemia due to severe spasm of the epicardial coronary arteries due to a catecholamine storm or direct damage of the myocyte by intense stimulation of the sympathetic nerves. This type of T wave abnormality can also be seen in patients with apical hypertrophic cardiomyopathy. (*Source*: Burch GE, Meyers R, Abildskov JA. A new electrocardiographic pattern observed in cerebrovascular accidents. *Circulation* 1954;9:720. Used with permission.)

IMITATORS OF MYOCARDIAL INFARCTION

Several conditions can simulate the electrocardiographic signs of myocardial infarction. The interpreter of the tracing *must* be knowledgeable about these masqueraders or a serious error can be made. The list of imitators includes the following:

The electrocardiograms of patients with pre-excitation of the ventricles (Wolff-Parkinson-White syndrome) may exhibit abnormal Q waves suggesting myocardial infarction (see Fig. 15-16).

The S-T segment displacement of acute pericarditis may be mistaken for myocardial infarction (see Fig. 17-2).

Abnormal Q waves, S-T segment displacement, and T waves simulating myocardial infarction related to coronary atherosclerotic heart disease may develop in the electrocardiograms of patients with myocarditis or myopericarditis.

Figure 15-16 This electrocardiogram, showing preexcitation of the ventricles and atrial fibrillation, was recorded from a 35-year-old man. This type of tracing is commonly mistaken for myocardial infarction and ventricular tachycardia. The P-R interval is 0.12 second and the duration of the QRS complex is 0.14 second. A delta wave is present. The spatial direction of the diagnostic cardiac vectors are shown in A through E. The large Q waves in lead II, III, aV_F imitate the Q wave abnormality of inferior infarction. The abnormal Q wave occurs because of the altered sequence of ventricular depolarization produced by a bypass tract. F. Atrial fibrillation. The ventricular rate is 290 complexes per minute. Such a tracing could be misinterpreted as being ventricular tachycardia. The congenital bypass tracts responsible for this condition occur most often in the absence of any other heart disease but the anomaly is more common in patients with Ebstein's anomaly and secundum atrial septal defect. (*Source:* Hurst JW. *Ventricular Electrocardiography*. New York: Gower Medical Publishing, 1991:11.35. The author, J.W.H., owns the copyright.)

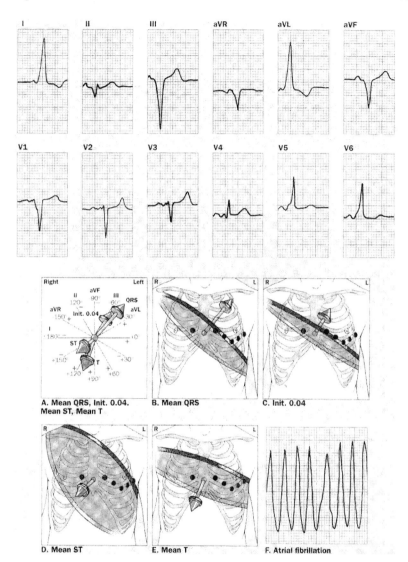

A. Mean QRS, Init. 0.04.
Mean ST, Mean T

B. Mean QRS

C. Init. 0.04

D. Mean ST

E. Mean T

F. Atrial fibrillation

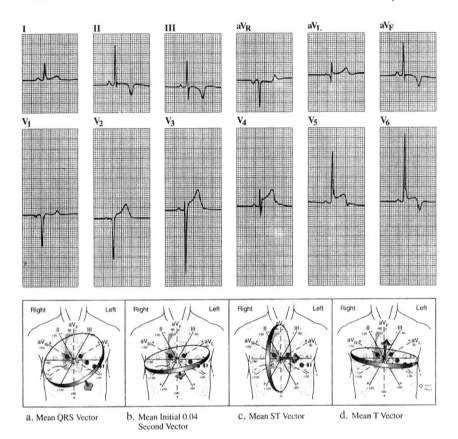

a. Mean QRS Vector   b. Mean Initial 0.04   c. Mean ST Vector   d. Mean T Vector
                          Second Vector

Figure 15-17 This electrocardiogram, showing the abnormalities associated with hypertrophic cardiomyopathy, was recorded from a 35-year-old man. Such abnormalities may be mistaken for those due to myocardial infarction. The P waves are normal and the P-R interval is 0.09 second. The duration of the QRS complex is 0.09 second. *a* through *d* illustrate the direction and relative size of the diagnostic cardiac vectors. The 12-lead QRS amplitude is 243 millimeters, indicating, along with the direction of the QRS vector, the likelihood of left ventricular hypertrophy. The absence of R waves in leads V_1 and V_2 could be caused by septal infarct or left ventricular hypertrophy. The mean S-T vector suggests lateral epicardial injury. The mean T vector suggests inferior ischemia. This type of tracing could be

The abnormal Q waves, S-T segment displacement, and T wave abnormalities of hypertrophic cardiomyopathy may simulate myocardial infarction (see Fig. 15-17).

Abnormal Q waves may occur in patients with dilated or restrictive cardiomyopathy (see Figs. 15-18 through 15-20).

Absent R waves in leads V_1–V_3 suggesting myocardial infarction may develop in patients with systolic pressure overload of the left ventricle, and large Q waves may develop in patients with diastolic pressure overload of the left ventricle (see Fig. 15-21).

Osborn waves may be mistaken for the abnormal S-T segments of infarction (see Fig. 23-3).

The noncoronary S-T segment abnormalities described by Brugada may be mistaken for those due to infarction (see Fig. 23-5).

---

caused by myocardial infarction, but because it was persistently the same and because left ventricular hypertrophy was likely, hypertrophic cardiomyopathy should be considered the best possibility. The presence of left ventricular hypertrophy in an electrocardiogram should be a red flag in any patient thought to have symptoms and signs of coronary atherosclerotic heart disease. Coronary atherosclerotic heart disease does not cause the electrocardiographic signs of left ventricular hypertrophy although the remaining viable myocytes may be hypertrophied. When the electrocardiographic signs of left ventricular hypertrophy are present in such a patient, it is wise to consider aortic valve stenosis or hypertension plus coronary atherosclerotic heart disease or to search for the clues for hypertrophic cardiomyopathy. (*Source*: Hurst JW. *Cardiovascular Diagnosis: The Initial Examination*. St. Louis: Mosby-Year Book, Inc, 1993:390. The author, J.W.H., owns the copyright.)

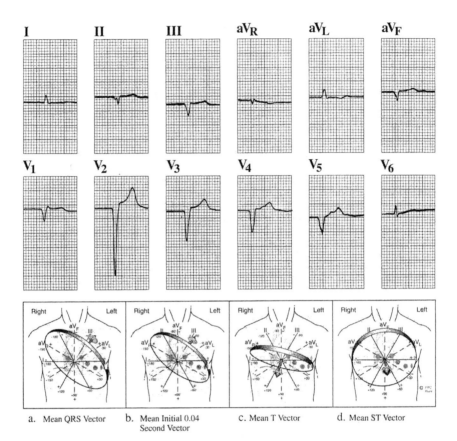

a. Mean QRS Vector   b. Mean Initial 0.04 Second Vector   c. Mean T Vector   d. Mean ST Vector

Figure 15-18 This electrocardiogram, showing abnormalities that imitate myocardial infarction, was recorded from a 69year-old woman with restrictive cardiomyopathy due to amyloid infiltration of the myocardium. No P waves are seen because there is junctional rhythm. The duration of the QRS complex is 0.08 second. The diagnostic cardiac vectors are illustrated in *a* through *d*. The 12-lead QRS amplitude is 76 millimeters and the initial 0.04 QRS vector is directed at $-58°$ in the frontal plane and posteriorly producing abnormal Q waves in leads II, III, aV_F, and $V_2–V_5$. Just as an increase in QRS amplitude is rarely caused by coronary diseases, a decrease in QRS amplitude is uncommonly due to coronary disease. This abnormality plus the strange and unusual direction of the initial 0.04 QRS vector should alert the interpreter to remember that there are numerous causes of "dead' or inert myocytes and that amyloid infiltration is one of them. (*Source*: Hurst JW. *Cardiovascular Diagnosis: The Initial Examination*. St. Louis: Mosby-Year Book, Inc, 1993:300. The author, J.W.H., owns the copyright.)

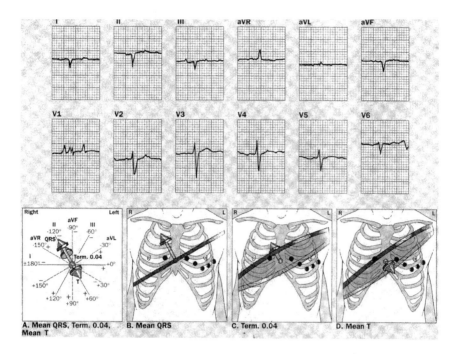

Figure 15-19 This electrocardiogram, showing abnormalities that imitate myocardial infarction, was recorded from a 31-year-old man with Friedreich's ataxia. Atrial tachycardia is present. (Note the two large P waves in lead V_1.) The duration of the QRS complex is 0.08 second. The spatial orientations of the diagnostic cardiac vectors are shown in A through D. The 12-lead QRS amplitude is 69 millimeters, and the mean QRS vector as well as the terminal 0.04 second QRS vector are directed in unusual directions. The low amplitude of the QRS complexes is uncommonly produced by coronary atherosclerotic coronary disease. When low amplitude of the QRS complexes is present in patients with coronary atherosclerotic heart disease, the patients commonly have "ischemic cardiomyopathy."

The low amplitude of the QRS complexes plus the unusual spatial directions of the mean QRS vector and the 0.04 second QRS vector should lead the interpreter to consider cardiomyopathy. In some instances the cardiomyopathy is part of a neurologic disease such as Friedreich's ataxia. (*Source*: Hurst JW. *Ventricular Electrocardiography*. New York: Gower Medical Publishing, 1991:11. 33. The author, J.W.H., owns the copyright.)

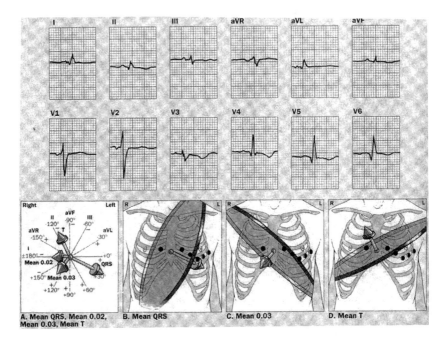

Figure 15-20 This electrocardiogram, showing abnormalities that imitate myocardial infarction, was recorded from a 43-year-old man with sarcoid heart disease. The P waves are abnormal; there is a left atrial abnormality. The P-R interval is 0.16 second and the duration of the QRS complexes is 0.11 second. The diagnostic cardiac vectors are illustrated in A through D. The QRS amplitude is 72 millimeters. The initial 0.02 and 0.03 second QRS vector are directed abnormally, producing abnormal Q waves in leads V_5 and V_6. The mean T vector is abnormal.

The low amplitude of the QRS complex plus the initial 0.03 second QRS abnormality should lead an interpreter to consider conditions other than coronary atherosclerotic heart disease as the cause of the abnormalities. In this case the abnormalities were caused by sarcoid heart disease. (*Source*: Hurst JW. *Ventricular Electrocardiography*. New York: Gower Medical Publishing, 1991: 11.34. The author, J.W.H., owns the copyright.)

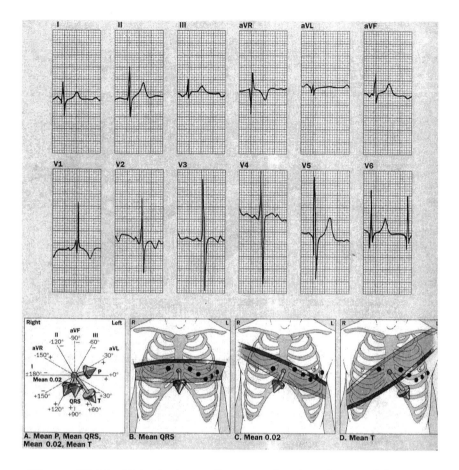

Figure 15-21 This electrocardiogram, showing abnormal Q waves that imitate myocardial infarction, was recorded from a 7-year-old boy with a large aortic septal defect due to congenital heart disease. The diagnostic cardiac vectors are illustrated in A through D. Note the direction of the P vector indicates the presence of lower atrial rhythm. The tracing shows biventricular hypertrophy due to diastolic overload. Note that the mean T vector is not directed opposite to the direction of the mean QRS vector. This tracing illustrates how large the initial QRS forces can be in patients with conditions that are caused by diastolic overload of the ventricles. The greatly enlarged surface area of the left ventricular endocardium is probably responsible for the large abnormal Q wave. (*Source*: Top: Hurst JW, Wenger NK (eds). *Electrocardiographic Interpretation*. New York: McGraw-Hill Book Company, 1963. Bottom: Hurst JW. *Ventricular Electrocardiography*. New York: Gower Medical Publishing, 1991: 11. 36. The author, J.W.H., owns the copyright.)

REFERENCES

1. Davies MJ. *Atlas of Coronary Artery Disease*. Philadelphia: Lippincott-Raven Publishers, 1998:1–161.

2. Harrison DC, Baim DS. Nonatherosclerotic causes of coronary heart disease. In: Hurst JW (ed-in-chief), *The Heart*, 7th ed., New York: McGraw-Hill, 1990;1130–1139.

3. Grant RP. *Clinical Electrocardiography: The Spatial Vector Approach*. New York: The Blakiston Division, McGraw-Hill Book Company, 1957:147–184.

4. Holland RP, Brooks H. TQ-ST segment mapping: Critical review and analysis of current concepts. *Am J Cardiol* 1977;40:110.

5. Hurst JW. *Ventricular Electrocardiography*. New York: Gower Medical Publishing, 1991:6.21.

6. Hurst JW, Pollak SJ, Brown CL, Lutz JF. Electrocardiographic signs suggesting inferior infarction associated with angiographic evidence of obstruction of the left anterior descending coronary artery or its branches. *Emory Univ J Med* 1988;2(3):170–176.

7. Perloff JK, Roberts WC, de Leon A, O'Doherty D. The distinctive electrocardiogram of Duchenne's progressive muscular dystrophy. *Am J Med* 1967 42:179–188.

Chapter 16

Electrocardiographic Abnormalities of the Conduction System of the Heart

GENERAL COMMENTS REGARDING THE ANATOMY AND FUNCTION OF THE CONDUCTION SYSTEM

The conduction system of the heart is one of the most ingenious parts of the human body. The purpose of these introductory remarks is to highlight some of the aspects of this remarkable system that must be understood by the clinician who interprets each electrocardiogram.

The sinus node, located in the upper part of the right atrium, is capable of spontaneous depolarization 60 to 80 times each minute (see Fig. 6-3A). The electrical impulse spreads through the right atrium before it reaches the left atrium. Investigators argue about the presence or absence of special cells that conduct the electrical activity in the atria, but there is no doubt that the depolarization process follows *preferential pathways* in the atria.

The electrical activity reaches the atrioventricular node (A-V node), which is located in the lower part of the right atrium (see Fig. 6-3A). The A-V node slows the conduction of electrical activity.

The His bundle joins the A-V node and conducts the electrical activity to the left and right ventricular conduction systems, where the speed of conduction is extremely rapid (see Fig. 6-3A).

The *left conduction system* is made up of a large fan-like structure that has three parts (see Fig. 6-3B). Tawara discovered that in 1906 (1). We do not know what all parts of the fan-like structure do, but we do know the following. A part of the fan directs the electrical impulse to the middle of the innermost part of the interventricular septum (see Fig. 6-3B). Another part, the left anterior-superior division, of the fan-like structure is directed anteriorly and superiorly (2), and still another part, the left posterior-superior division, is directed inferiorly and posteriorly (see Fig. 6-3B) (3). The *right bundle* passes down the anterior part of the interventricular septum sending small branches to the septal area (see Fig. 6-3C). It then curves upward in the right ventricle. The left and right conduction systems are completed when the small distal branches of the system divide into the Purkinje fibers that have an intimate relationship with the ventricular myocytes.

The electrical charges that stimulate the myocyctes set in motion a different ionic chain of events that causes the cells to contract. The myocytes slow electrical conduction and create the deflection seen in the electrocardiogram.

Abnormalities of the atrial and ventricular conduction system, such as sinus arrest, sinoatrial block, and varying degrees of atrioventricular block, are usually discussed in connection with cardiac arrhythmias. This chapter deals with nonarrhythmic abnormalities of the left and right ventricular conduction systems that are recognized by identifying alterations in the P waves, the QRS complexes, and their associated S-T and T waves.

ADDITIONAL COMMENTS AND HYPOTHESES REGARDING THE ROLE OF THE CONDUCTION SYSTEM IN THE TRANSMISSION OF ELECTRICAL ACTIVITY

Our knowledge of the conduction system and its influence on the sequence of depolarization of the heart is still evolving. It is clear today that previous discussions of the electrocardiographic abnormalities caused by conduction defects were grossly oversimplified. The following discussion and hypothesis are based on the correlation of the electrocardiographic abnormalities with other clinical data and deductive reasoning. Many of the comments are presented as reasonable assumptions but are not always based on proven scientific facts. With this caveat, I offer the following comments.

The left ventricular conduction system is not a bundle. The word bundle conjures up the image of a strand or a rope. The system is composed of a fan-like structure that is divided into three parts (see Fig. 6-3B). This being true, I will no longer refer to the left ventricular conduction *system* as a bundle.

The right ventricular conduction system is a bundle; there is no fan-like structure on the right side.

The interventricular septum in the adult is that part of the left ventricle that is located anteriorly; the right ventricle simply rides the left ventricle (see Fig. 6-1B).

The initial 0.01 second of the QRS complex is normally produced by stimulation of the myocytes located in the middle of the left side of the interventricular septum. Normally, the depolarization of the interventricular septum produces an electrical force that is directed from left-to-right and anteriorly. The exact direction of the vector representing this force is influenced considerably by the precise location of the heart in the chest, but the depolarization of the septum is commonly directed to the right and anteriorly.

The initial 0.04 second of the QRS complex is normally produced by the depolarization of the endocardial surfaces of both ventricles, including the interventricular septum. In the adult, the mean vector representing the initial 0.04 second of the QRS complex is usually directed to the left, inferiorly, and approximately parallel with the frontal plane.

The electrical forces that create the middle part of the QRS complex in the normal adult are produced by an increasing number of left ventricular forces and a dwindling number of right ventricular forces. A mean vector representing these forces in the adult is usually directed to the left, inferiorly and slightly posteriorly. This occurs because the normal left ventricle of the adult is thicker than the right ventricle. The forces are directed posteriorly because the left posterior-inferior branch of the left conduction system conducts the electrical activity to the posterior portion of the left ventricle.

The terminal 0.01 to 0.02 second of the QRS complex of the normal adult is produced by the depolarization of the superior portion of the left ventricle. The exact direction of the vector representing this force is influenced considerably by the location of the heart in the chest, but it is commonly directed to the left and posteriorly.

The duration of the normal QRS complex: The duration of the normal QRS complex in the adult is usually less than 0.10 second.

Hypertrophy of the left or right ventricles may prolong the QRS complex slightly, rarely more than 0.01 second.

When there is damage to the left anterior superior division or the left posterior inferior division of the conduction system, the QRS duration may not be prolonged more than 0.01 second.

Damage to a part of the proximal portion of the left conduction system or to the right bundle produces prolongation of the QRS complexes to 0.12 second.

When the QRS duration is 0.14 or 0.16 second or more, it is necessary to postulate that a major part of the blockade of the conduction system is located in the distal part of the left ventricular conduction system or the distal part of the right bundle. This hints of a Purkinje-myocyte block. Such a finding should alert the clinician that this is not an ordinary uncomplicated left ventricular conduction system block or simple uncomplicated right bundle branch block. When the QRS duration is greater than 0.12 second, it is not uncommon for there to be ventricular dilatation of the left or right ventricles in addition to the block, or some other condition that damages the entire heart such as hypothermia, various drugs, electrolyte abnormalities, or poison. Because dilatation of the left or right ventricles is the most comon additional factor causing a QRS duration of 0.14 to 0.16 second, it leads one to wonder if dilatation of a ventricle can stretch the distal parts of the conduction system so the system cannot conduct properly, or if there is damage to the myocytes so the Purkinje-myocyte union is faulty. It is not uncommon, for instance, to observe the QRS duration of 0.10 second associated with right or left ventricular hypertrophy and dilatation to gradually increase until the QRS duration is 0.14 second in duration. The increase in QRS duration in such cases is more likely due to the dilatation of the ventricles than to concentric hypertrophy of the ventricles.

The direction of the mean QRS vector: The mean QRS vector may not shift very much when uncomplicated ventricular conduction abnormalities develop. This is because the direction of the mean QRS vector is greatly influenced by electrical forces that produce the initial and middle portion of the QRS complex. The terminal forces produced by ventricular depolarization point toward the ventricle in which depolarization is delayed. Accordingly, the mean QRS vector may not shift more than 40° to 60° from its pre-block position. Therefore, "left or right" axis deviation of the mean QRS vector is not an essential part of the criteria for the identification of ventricular conduction abnormalities. The direction of the terminal 0.02 to

0.04 second vector is, however, very important for it identifies the right or left ventricle in which the delay of the depolarization is occurring.

When the mean QRS vector is directed more than 40° to 60° from the normal pre-block position, one should postulate that a complicated type of block exists; it is not a simple uncomplicated block in the proximal portion of the left conduction system or in the proximal part of the right bundle. Because one does not always have a pre-block electrocardiogram and thus cannot make the comparison, one can assume that the mean QRS vector of *most* normal adults is directed at +30° to +60° in the frontal plane and about 45° posteriorly.* Therefore, when the duration of the QRS complexes is 0.12 second or greater, and the mean QRS vector is directed more than −30° to the left or more than +120° to the right, the conduction abnormality is not an ordinary, uncomplicated, ventricular conduction abnormality.

Anyone who is seriously interested in electrocardiography will encounter tracings with conduction system abnormalities that cannot be explained. The interpreter who knows basic principles will be in a better position to explain them than the interpreter who uses the memory system of interpretation. Still, there are tracings that no one can explain.

Conventional thought holds that the electrocardiogram gives no information about the contractile ability of the heart. As stated many times in this book, the basic mechanism that is responsible for the electrical activity is different from the basic mechanism that produces contraction of the myocytes. The extreme example of the separation of these two mechanisms is seen in patients with electrical-mechanical dissociation. The heart in such patients is not contracting properly yet the electrocardiogram reveals P, QRS, and T waves. Also we

---

* The normal range for the direction of the mean QRS vector is discussed in Chapter 12; the range itself is much wider than +30° to +60°. However, it is true that the direction of the mean QRS vector of *most* normal adults is between +30° to +60° in the frontal plane.

observe the return of P waves in patients whose atrial fibrillation reverts to normal rhythm, but this does not guarantee that atrial contraction has returned to normal. These examples serve to support the notion that the electrocardiogram does not yield information about the functional status of the heart. Despite this conventional thinking, and the examples cited, I believe there may be several electrocardiographic abnormalities that correlate with poor ejection fractions or other measurements of poor cardiac function. For example, my colleagues at Emory and I studied patients who had total correction of tetralogy of Fallot early in their life, but later had signs of right ventricular dysfunction suggested clinically and proved by magnetic resonance imaging (4). We discovered we could predict which patients had right ventricular dysfunction by identifying a right conduction system abnormality in which the QRS duration was 0.14 second or more and the mean QRS vector was directed toward the northwest quadrant of the hexaxial reference system.

A left atrial abnormality may develop transiently during acute myocardial infarction. One wonders if it signifies a transient rise in left ventricular diastolic pressure.

At present many interpreters and outdated computers state only that tracings reveal either left or right bundle branch block. This, of course, is obviously inadequate because our current knowledge goes far beyond such simple designations.

CLASSIFICATION OF VENTRICULAR CONDUCTION SYSTEM ABNORMALITIES

Abnormalities of the Left Ventricular Conduction System

Abnormalities of the left ventricular system can be categorized as follows:

Left ventricular conduction delay
Left anterior-superior division block (2)
Left posterior-inferior division block (3)

Uncomplicated proximal left ventricular conduction system block, formerly referred to as uncomplicated left
bundle branch block

Complicated left conduction system block; the system is
said to be complicated when one or more of the following abnormalities is present: the QRS duration
is greater than 0.12 second, the mean QRS vector is
directed more than −30° to the left, the mean QRS
vector is directed to the left and anterior, the mean
T vector is caused by a primary T wave abnormality,
or the mean S-T segment vector is caused by a primary S-T segment abnormality (5)

Abnormalities of the Right Ventricular Conduction System

Abnormalities of the right ventricular conduction system can
be categorized as follows:

Right ventricular conduction delay.

Uncomplicated right bundle branch block.

Complicated right bundle branch block; the system is said
to be complicated when one or more of the following
abnormalities is present: the QRS duration is
greater than 0.12 second, the mean QRS vector is
directed more than +120° to the right, the mean
QRS vector is directed to the left and anteriorly, abnormal Q waves are present, a primary T wave abnormality is present, or a primary S-T segment abnormality is apparent (5)

Nondescript Ventricular Conduction System Abnormalities

Ventricular conduction abnormalities may be seen that do not
fit neatly into the classification discussed above; they are clas-
sified as nondescript and are often seen in patients with diseases of the myocardium or in patients with congenital heart
disease.

DISCUSSIONS AND EXAMPLES OF SPECIFIC LEFT VENTRICULAR CONDUCTION SYSTEM ABNORMALITIES

Left Ventricular Conduction Delay

Left ventricular conduction system delay is said to be present when the duration of the QRS complexes is normal but there are other abnormalities similar to those characteristic of uncomplicated proximal left ventricular conduction system block in which the QRS duration is 0.12 second or longer.

The initial 0.01 to 0.02 sec QRS vector is directed to the left and posteriorly. This results in the absence of Q waves in leads I and V_6 and no R wave, or a very small R wave in lead V_1. This suggests that the depolarization of the septum is reversed, as it is with uncomplicated proximal left ventricular conduction system block.

The terminal 0.02 to 0.04 second QRS vector is directed to the left and posteriorly, as it is in uncomplicated proximal left ventricular conduction system block.

This abnormality has not been studied in an organized fashion, but it could be the result of damage to the middle portion of the inner aspect of the interventricular septum. This could be the result of myocardial damage due to coronary atherosclerotic heart disease, localized infiltrative disease, or myocyte replacement with fibrosis in patients with cardiomyopathy. I have seen such tracings in young healthy patients who have no other evidence of heart disease, suggesting, but not proving, that in some patients the abnormality could be a congenital variant of the conduction system.

An electrocardiogram depicting left ventricular conduction delay is shown in Figure 16-1.

Left Anterior-Superior Division Block

The duration of the QRS complexes is never more than 0.10 second.

The initial 0.01 second QRS vector is usually directed to the right, inferiorly, and anteriorly because the ini-

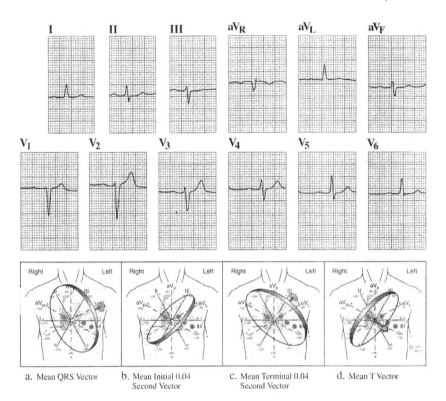

I II III aV~R~ aV~L~ aV~F~

V~1~ V~2~ V~3~ V~4~ V~5~ V~6~

a. Mean QRS Vector   b. Mean Initial 0.04   c. Mean Terminal 0.04   d. Mean T Vector
                         Second Vector   Second Vector

Figure 16-1 This electrocardiogram, showing left ventricular conduction delay, was recorded from a 67-year-old man with coronary arteriographic evidence of obstruction coronary atherosclerosis. The P waves are normal and the P-R interval is 0.24 second, signifying first-degree atrioventricular block. The duration of the QRS complexes is 0.09 to 0.10 second. In *a* through *d*, the mean QRS and T vectors are normal. The mean initial 0.04 QRS vector is directed more posteriorly than usual. The mean initial 0.01 vector is directed to the left and parallel with the frontal plane. There are no Q waves in leads I and V~6~ and there is a very small R wave in lead V~1~. The duration of the QRS complexes is 0.10 second. The long P-R interval, a QRS duration of 0.10 second, and no Q waves in leads I and V~6~ with a very small R wave at lead V~1~ leads one to believe the tracing is abnormal due to first-degree atrioventricular block and left ventricular conduction delay. Left ventricular delay may develop in patial part of the left anterior-superior division of the left ventricular conduction system commonly curves slightly to the right before it curves superiorly and anteriorly (2).

When the left anterior-superior division of the left ventricular conduction system is damaged, the mean QRS vector shifts so that it is directed at $-30°$ or more to the left and posteriorly.

This type of QRS vector may be associated with left ventricular hypertrophy, but left ventricular hypertrophy is not the primary cause of the conduction abnormality. Remember, most patients with left ventricular hypertrophy do not have abnormal left axis deviation of the mean QRS vector.

Left anterior-superior division block occurs with increasing frequency as individuals become older. The cause of this phenomenon is not known, but it may be related to apoptosis of a part of the left ventricular conduction system.

Left anterior-superior division block may occur without other evidence of heart disease.

An electrocardiogram depicting left anterior-superior division block is shown in Figure 16-2.

Left Posterior-Inferior Division Block

Left posterior-inferior division block occurs less often than left anterior-superior division block (4). This is thought to be the case because the blood supply to the left posterior-inferior divi-

---

tients with coronary atherosclerotic heart disease, but there may be other causes such as cardiomyopathy. The condition has not been studied adequately, and at present the observation must be interpreted within the context of other clinical data. (*Source*: Hurst JW. *Cardiovascular Diagnosis: The Initial Examination*. St. Louis: Mosby-Year Book, Inc, 1993:310. The author, J.W.H., owns the copyright.)

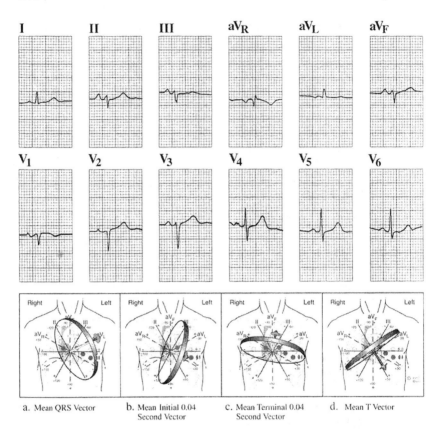

a. Mean QRS Vector   b. Mean Initial 0.04   c. Mean Terminal 0.04   d. Mean T Vector
Second Vector   Second Vector

Figure 16-2 This electrocardiogram, showing left anterior-superior division block, was recorded from a 59-year-old asymptomatic woman. There was no other evidence of heart disease. The tracing had not changed in nearly two decades. The P waves are normal and the P-R interval is 0.14 second. The duration of the QRS complexes is 0.08 second. In a, the mean QRS vector is directed about $-28°$ to $-30°$ to the left and about $50°$ to $60°$ posteriorly. The direction of the initial 0.04 QRS vector is shown in b. In c, the mean terminal 0.04 QRS vector is directed at about $-80°$ in the frontal plane and more than $40°$ posteriorly. In d, the mean T vector is directed at $+55°$ in the frontal plane and $5°$ anteriorly. The direction of the mean QRS vector at $-28°$ to $-30°$ with a normal QRS duration signifies the presence of left anterior-superior division block. The direction of the

sion is derived from the left anterior descending coronary artery plus the branches off the right coronary artery, whereas the blood supply to the left anterior-superior division is derived from the left anterior descending artery (3).

When the posterior-inferior division is damaged, the terminal forces of the QRS complexes are directed to the right. The duration of the QRS complexes remain normal, although they may be slightly longer than they were prior to the block. This causes the mean QRS vector to be directed more than $+120°$ to the right and posteriorly, producing S waves in leads I and V_1-V_6 (3).

The tracing may simulate the abnormalities seen in right ventricular delay, except in the latter, the terminal forces are directed anteriorly rather than posteriorly as they are with left-posterior-inferior division block.

It is difficult to make a definite identification of isolated left posterior-inferior division block except when the clinical context includes a previous normal tracing and other clinical abnormalities that support the diagnosis of coronary disease or some other disease, such as cardiomyopathy, where it is reasonable to assume that the left posterior-inferior division could develop.

As discussed later in this chapter, left posterior-inferior division block may occur when there is right bundle branch

---

ventricular gradient is borderline, suggesting the possibility of a primary T wave abnormality.

This patient exhibited no other evidence of heart disease and the abnormality had been present for almost 20 years. Was the abnormality a variant that was congenital in origin? This type of conduction defect occurs more commonly in older patients, suggesting that apoptosis of some of the cells in the conduction system is the cause. Finally, the conduction defect occurs in some patients with left ventricular hypertrophy, but it is not due to the hypertrophic muscle itself. (*Source*: Hurst JW. *Cardiovascular Diagnosis: The Initial Examination*. St. Louis: Mosby-Year Book, Inc, 1993:316. The author, J.W.H., owns the copyright.)

block. In such cases the mean QRS vector is directed father to the right than 120° (see Fig. 16-8). Even in these cases there are other causes of a far-right mean QRS vector and the identification of additional left posterior-inferior division block is difficult to make with certainty.

Uncomplicated Proximal Left Ventricular Conduction System Block

Uncomplicated proximal left ventricular conduction system block is said to be present when the following electrocardiographic abnormalities are present.

> The duration of the QRS complexes is 0.12 second. This determination should be made by viewing the complexes rather than accepting the computer readout of the measurement.
>
> The mean QRS vector may be directed 30° to 60° to the left of its pre-block position. It is usually directed at about +20° to +60°, but it is never directed more than −30° to the left. It is always directed posteriorly.
>
> The initial 0.01 to 0.02 second QRS vector is directed to the left and posteriorly because depolarization of the septum is from right to left and posteriorly rather than from left to right and anteriorly, as it is normally. This occurs because small branches off the intact right bundle conduct the electricity to the septum, causing its depolarization. Accordingly, there are no Q waves in leads I and V_6, and the R wave is absent or small in lead V_1.
>
> The terminal 0.02 to 0.04 second QRS vector is directed to the left and posteriorly toward the left ventricle.
>
> The mean spatial S-T segment vector is usually directed within 30° to 60° of the mean spatial T vector (5). Like the T wave, it is due to the forces of repolariza-

tion. It is referred to as a secondary S-T segment vector. As will be discussed later, when the mean S-T vector is large and is directed more than 60° or so away from the mean T vector, the conduction defect has become complicated because there may be a separate cause for the S-T segment displacement. Under these circumstances the S-T segment displacement is referred to as a primary S-T segment abnormality (5).

The mean spatial T wave vector is directed away from the mean QRS vector. Therefore, it is usually directed to the right and anteriorly. The abnormal looking T wave may be normal for the obviously abnormal QRS complex because the direction of the repolarization process is predetermined by the direction of the depolarization process. Therefore, the challenge is to determine whether the T waves are abnormal looking only because of the QRS conduction abnormality or whether they are abnormal because a separate abnormality is causing the T wave changes. Therefore, when possible the ventricular gradient should be constructed. When the ventricular gradient is normal, one can assume that the abnormal-looking T waves are actually normal for that particular QRS abnormality. In such patients the abnormal-looking T waves changes are referred to as secondary T wave changes. When the ventricular gradient is abnormal, a primary T wave abnormality is said to be present. This signifies that a condition has developed in the myocardium that has altered the direction of the repolarization process over and beyond the changes expected because the repolarization sequence has been predetermined by the QRS conduction abnormality. When this occurs, the uncomplicated left bundle branch block has become complicated.

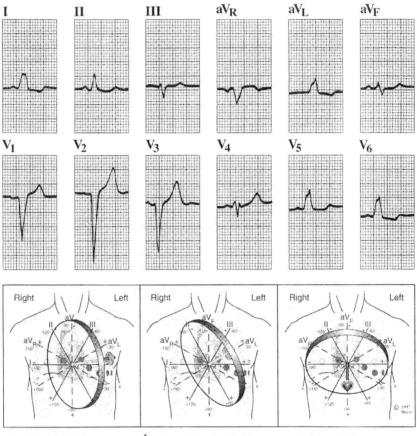

a. Mean QRS Vector   b. Mean Terminal 0.04   c. Mean T Vector
                             Second Vector

Figure 16-3   This electrocardiogram, showing uncomplicated proximal left ventricular system block, was recorded from a patient who had no other signs of heart disease. This abnormality was previously called left bundle branch block. The P waves are normal and the P-R interval is 0.14 second. The duration of the QRS complexes is 0.12 to 0.13 second. In *a*, the mean QRS vector is directed at −8° in the frontal plane and about 50° posteriorly. In *b*, the mean terminal 0.04 QRS vector is directed −3° in the frontal plane and about 40° posteriorly. In *c*, the mean T vector is directed at +90° in the frontal plane and about 85° anteriorly. The ventricular gradient is normal.

The cause of the secondary S-T and T wave changes is not known when there is uncomplicated proximal left ventricular conduction system block, but they are likely produced because uncomplicated left ventricular conduction block alters the sequence of left ventricular contraction and, by doing so, decreases the true transmyocardial pressure gradient. This, in turn, causes the repolarization process to be directed from endocardium to epicardium, which reverses the direction of the repolarization forces (5). The S-T segment in such a situation is due to repolarization forces and is actually part of the T wave. This explanation is supported by the observation that ventricular pacemakers seem to alter the sequence of contraction in patients with idiopathic hypertrophic subaortic stenosis and in some patients with dilated cardiomyopathy.

Uncomplicated proximal left ventricular conduction system block may be produced by coronary atherosclerotic heart disease; cardiomyopathy or generalized myocardial damage from any of many causes; aortic valve disease from any cause; mitral valve disease, such as mitral valve annulus disease; primary disease of the conduction system; various drugs; and surgical procedures.

An electrocardiogram depicting uncomplicated proximal left ventricular conduction system block is shown in Figure 16–3.

Uncomplicated proximal left ventricular conduction system block may be caused by coronary atherosclerotic heart disease, cardiomyopathy, aortic and/or mitral valve disease with annular calcification, primary disease of the conduction system, and unknown causes in which apoptosis is a possibility. (*Source*: Top: Stein E. *Electrocardiographic Interpretation: A Self-Study Approach to Clinical Electrocardiology*. Philadelphia: Lea & Febiger, 1991:432. Used with permission. Bottom: Hurst JW. *Cardiovascular Diagnosis: The Initial Examination*. St. Louis: Mosby-Year Book, Inc, 1993:330. The author, J.W.H., owns the copyright.)

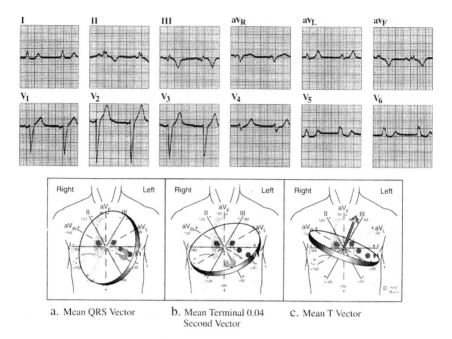

a. Mean QRS Vector   b. Mean Terminal 0.04   c. Mean T Vector
                             Second Vector

Figure 16-4 This electrocardiogram, showing proximal left ventricular conduction system block and inferior myocardial ischemia, was recorded from a 59-year-old man who had experienced an inferioposterior myocardial infarction. The mean P vector is directed at $+90°$ in the frontal plane and about 40° posteriorly. The negative P waves in leads V_1-V_3 indicate a left atrial abnormality. The duration of the QRS complexes is 0.12 second. In a, the mean QRS vector is directed at $+20°$ in the frontal plane and almost 70° posteriorly. In b, the mean terminal 0.04 second QRS vector is directed at $+70°$ in the frontal plane and 50° posteriorly. In c, the mean T vector is directed at $-70°$ in the frontal plane. It is not possible to determine accurately the anterior-posterior direction of the mean T vector because all of the T waves are upright in the leads V_1-V_6. However, it is possible to state that the T vector is directed about 30° or more anteriorly. The ventricular gradient is definitely abnormal; it is directed at approximately $-40°$.

The primary T wave abnormality is caused by the inferior-posterior epicardial ischemia associated with myocardial infarction. (*Source*: Top: The electrocardiogram is from Hurst JW, Woodson GC

Complicated Left Ventricular Conduction System Block

Uncomplicated left ventricular conduction system block becomes complicated when the duration of the QRS complex is longer than 0.12 to 0.13 second, when the mean QRS vector is directed more than −30° to the left, or is directed anteriorly rather than posteriorly, and when the mean S-T or T vectors are not directed as they are in patients with uncomplicated proximal left ventricular conduction system block (5).

When uncomplicated or complicated proximal left ventricular conduction sytem block is present, the interventricular septum is depolarized from right to left and posteriorly; this usually prevents the development of abnormal initial QRS forces (abnormal Q wave) due to myocardial infarction. Because abnormal Q waves due to myocardial infarction cannot usually be identified when there is left ventricular conduction system block, it is essential for an interpreter to be able to recognize primary S-T segment abnormalities and primary T wave abnormalities in the electrocardiogram (5).

An example of complicated left ventricular conduction system block due to a primary T wave abnormality is depicted in Figure 16-4. Note that the direction of the ventricular gradient is abnormal; this signifies that a primary T wave abnormality is present.

Complicated Left Ventricular Conduction System Block with Intact Septal Depolarization

The initial septal depolarization in these patients is intact but the QRS duration is abnormally long. Presumably, in such pa-

---

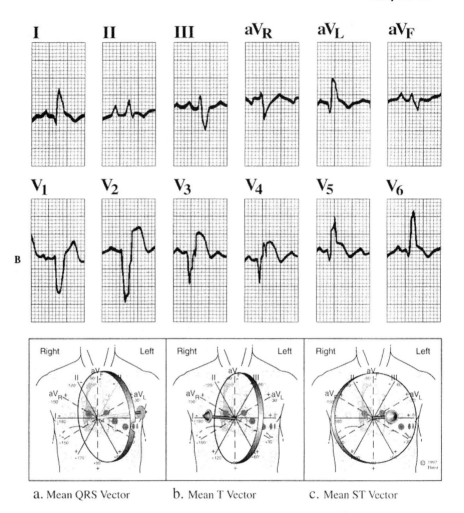

a. Mean QRS Vector   b. Mean T Vector   c. Mean ST Vector

Figure 16-5 This electrocardiogram, showing left conduction system block with intact septal depolarization, was recorded from a patient with an extensive anterolateral myocardial infarction. The P waves are normal and the P-R interval is 0.14 second. The duration of the QRS complexes is 0.12 second. The mean initial 0.03 second QRS vector is directed to the right and anteriorly. This produces Q waves in leads I and V6 and an R wave in lead V_1 and V_2. Normal depolarization of the septum seems to be intact, because ordinarily,

tients, the conduction defect is located in the more distal branches of the left conduction system.

An example of complicated left ventricular conduction system block with intact septal depolarization is shown in Figure 16-5. In the example shown, the conduction abnormality is also complicated because a primary S-T segment abnormality is present.

Complicated Left Ventricular Conduction System Block Due to Additional Left Anterior-Superior Division Block

Complicated proximal left ventricular conduction system block due to additional left anterior-superior division block can be identified when the following abnormalities are present:

---

with proximal left ventricular conduction system block (formerly called left bundle branch block), the depolarization of the septum is from right to left which eliminates the Q waves at lead I and V_6 and the small R wave at V_1. In a, the mean QRS vector is directed at about $-15°$ in the frontal plane and about $60°-70°$ posteriorly. In b, the mean T vector is directed at about $-170°$ in the frontal plane and about $40°$ anteriorly. The ventricular gradient is directed abnormally, signifying the presence of a primary T wave abnormality. In c, the huge mean S-T vector is directed at $-5°$ in the frontal plane and at least $85°$ anteriorly. The ST-T angle is about $55°$ but the S-T segment vector is extremely large, indicating the presence of a primary S-T segmental abnormality. The left ventricular system block in this patient was probably located in the distal portion of the conduction system because the depolarization of the septum is intact. In addition, the directions of the mean S-T and T vectors indicate extensive anterolateral myocardial infarction. (*Source*: Top: Hurst JW, Woodson GC Jr. *Atlas of Spatial Vector Electrocardiography*. New York: The Blakiston Company, Inc, 1951:183. The author, J.W.H., owns the copyright. Bottom: The diagrams shown in *A*, *B*, and *C* are from Hurst JW. *Cardiovascular Diagnosis: The Initial Examination*. St. Louis: Mosby-Year Book, Inc, 1993:350. The author, J.W.H., owns the copyright.)

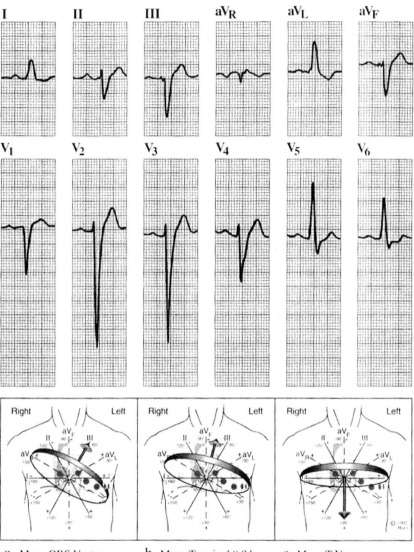

a. Mean QRS Vector

b. Mean Terminal 0.04 Second Vector

c. Mean T Vector

The duration of the QRS complexes is 0.12 second or more.

The initial 0.01 to 0.02 sec QRS vector is directed to the left and posteriorly because the depolarization of the septum is directed from right to left and posteriorly rather than being directed from left to right and anteriorly as it is normally.

The mean QRS vector may be directed more than −30° to the left and posteriorly. Presumably this occurs because the left anterior-superior division of the conduction system is also disrupted. This permits the

---

Figure 16-6 This electrocardiogram, showing complicated left ventricular conduction system block plus left anterior superior division block, was recorded from a 43-year-old man with acromegaly and a large heart. The P waves are normal and the P-R interval is 0.20 second. The duration of the QRS complexes is 0.15 to 0.16 second. This degree of prolongation is another reason this tracing does not show simple uncomplicated left ventricular conduction system block. In *a*, the mean QRS vector is directed at −60° in the frontal plane and at least 30° posteriorly. The far-left direction of the mean QRS vector signifies the presence of additional left anterior superior direction block. In *b*, the mean initial 0.04 second QRS vector is directed at −75° in the frontal plane and 30° posteriorly. In *c*, the mean T vector is directed at +90° in the frontal plane and more than 20° anteriorly. The ventricular gradient is at about 0° in the frontal plane, which is probably abnormal. This electrocardiogram shows proximal left ventricular conduction system block complicated by QRS prolongation beyond 0.12 second and additional left anterior-superior division block. These abnormalities commonly signify the presence of a large left ventricle due to left ventricular disease.

Patients with acromegaly may have cardiomyopathy. They also have a greater than average likelihood of having coronary atherosclerotic heart disease. The patient discussed here was believed to have cardiomyopathy, but coronary disease was not definitely excluded. (*Source*: Hurst JW. *Cardiovascular Diagnosis. The Initial Examination*. St. Louis: Mosby-Year Book, Inc, 1993:356. The author, J.W.H., owns the copyright.)

posterior-inferior division of the conduction system
to transmit electrical activity to posterior and inferior portions of the heart and beyond.

The mean terminal 0.04 sec QRS vector is directed far to
the left and posteriorly.

The mean S-T vector is usually directed within 30 to 60°
of the mean T vector. It is usually due to repolarization forces and is part of the T. When the mean ST
vector is large and is directed more than 60° away
from the mean T vector it may be due to epicardial
injury such as occurs with myocardial infarction.

When the ventricular gradient is abnormal, a primary T
wave abnormality is thought to be present.

Complicated proximal left ventricular conduction system
block due to additional left anterior-superior division block
may be caused by coronary atherosclerotic heart disease, cardiomyopathy, aortic and mitral valve disease with a large left
ventricle, primary disease of the conduction system, certain
drugs, or cardiac surgery.

An example of complicated left ventricular conduction
system block due to additional left anterior-superior division
block is shown in Figure 16-6.

DISCUSSION AND EXAMPLES OF SPECIFIC
RIGHT VENTRICULAR CONDUCTION
SYSTEM ABNORMALITIES

Right Ventricular Conduction Delay

Right ventricular conduction delay is said to be present when
the duration of the QRS complex is normal but other abnormalities are present that are similar to those that are characteristic of uncomplicated right bundle branch block.

The duration of the QRS complexes is 0.10 second or less.
The measurement should be made by viewing the

complexes rather than accepting the readout produced by a computer. As time passes, the QRS duration may become longer than normal in some patients. Should the duration become 0.12 second, the tracing is labeled as right bundle branch block.

The mean initial 0.01 to 0.02 second QRS vector is directed almost normally.

The mean QRS vector is directed to the right and anteriorly. It is rarely directed more than $+120°$ to the right. The mean QRS vector may be directed more than $+120°$ to the right when the condition is caused by, or is associated with, a large right ventricle.

The vector representing the mean terminal 0.02 to 0.04 second portion of the QRS complex is directed to the right and anteriorly or parallel with the frontal plane. It is directed toward the right ventricle. This produces an S wave in leads I and V_6 and a tall terminal R-prime wave in lead V_1.

The mean S-T vector is directed relatively parallel with the mean T vector and is caused by the repolarization process.

The mean T vector may be directed to the left and posteriorly. It tends to be directed away from the right ventricle.

Right ventricular conduction delay is commonly observed in patients with ostium secundum atrial septal defect. In such cases it masks the findings that could be theoretically produced by diastolic pressure overload of the right ventricle. Right ventricular conduction delay may also be produced by acute pulmonary embolism and may occur in patients who have no other evidence of heart disease.

An electrocardiogram showing right ventricular conduction delay is similar to the tracing showing uncomplicated right bundle branch block, except the duration of the QRS complex is less than 0.12 second (see Fig. 16-7).

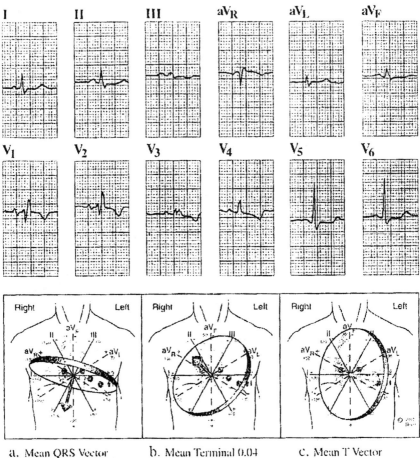

a. Mean QRS Vector   b. Mean Terminal 0.04   c. Mean T Vector
                     Second Vector

Figure 16-7 This electrocardiogram, showing uncomplicated right bundle branch block, was recorded from a 65-year-old woman with an ostium secundum atrial septal defect. The P waves are normal and the P-R interval is 0.14 second. The duration of the QRS complexes is 0.12 second. In *a*, the mean QRS vector is directed at +105° in the frontal plane and about 15° to 20° anteriorly. In *b*, the mean terminal 0.04 second QRS vector is directed at −135° in the frontal plane and about 60° anteriorly. In *c*, the mean T vector is directed at +10° in the frontal plane and 60°−70° posteriorly. The ventricular

Uncomplicated Right Bundle Branch Block

Uncomplicated right bundle branch block is believed to be present when the following abnormalities are identified in the electrocardiogram.

The duration of the QRS complex is 0.12 second. The measurement should be made by viewing the QRS complexes instead of accepting the computer readout.

The initial 0.01 to 0.02 second QRS vector is directed almost normally.

The mean QRS vector is directed inferiorly and anteriorly toward the right ventricle. It is rarely directed more than $+120°$ to the right.

The mean spatial S-T vector is directed within 30° to 60° of the mean T vector. It is caused by repolarization of the ventricles and is referred to as a secondary S-T segment change.

The mean T vector is directed to the left and posteriorly away from the right ventricle. When there is uncom-

---

gradient is normal. The duration of the QRS complexes is 0.12 second in this tracing. Along with the secondary T wave abnormality, this tracing is designated as one exhibiting uncomplicated right bundle branch block. *When the duration of the QRS complexes is 0.08 to 0.11 second, a similar tracing is referred to as exhibiting right ventricular conduction delay.* Although such a tracing can occur in the absence of other signs of heart disease, it is wise to consider diastolic overload of the right ventricle as occurs with ostium secundum atrial septal defect. As discussed in Chapter 14, the theoretical signs of diastolic overload of the right ventricle are masked by the electrocardiographic signs of right ventricular conduction delay. Right bundle branch block can also occur secondary to coronary atherosclerotic heart disease, cardiomyopathy, and longstanding right ventricular hypertrophy of any cause. (*Source*: Hurst JW. *Cardiovascular Diagnosis: The Initial Examination.* St. Louis: Mosby-Year Book, Inc, 1993:324. The author, J.W.H., owns the copyright.)

plicated right bundle branch block, the ventricular gradient is normal. Accordingly, the abnormal-appearing T waves and mean T vector are referred to as secondary T wave changes. Remember, the direction of the depolarization process predetermines the direction of repolarization process. Accordingly, the abnormal-looking T waves are the result of the abnormal sequence of depolarization rather than being due to a primary cause of altered repolarization.

The physiological reason for secondary S-T and T wave changes is not known, but they may occur because the abnormal sequence of depolarization alters the sequence of contraction of the right ventricle and the usual transmyocardial pressure gradient does not develop during systole. Accordingly, the direction of repolarization in the right ventricle becomes reversed.

Uncomplicated right bundle branch block can be caused by coronary atherosclerotic heart disease; cardiomyopathy; longstanding right ventricular hypertrophy or dilatation from any of several causes, including pulmonary valve stenosis, tetralogy of Fallot, secundum atrial septal defect, or pulmonary hypertension of any cause, including pulmonary emboli and primary pulmonary hypertension; cardiac surgery; certain drugs; and primary disease of the conduction system.

An example of uncomplicated right bundle branch block is depicted in Figure 16–7.

Complicated Right Bundle Branch Block

Complicated right bundle branch block is believed to be present when one or more of the following abnormalities are identified in the electrocardiogram.

The duration of the QRS complex is greater than 0.12 second.

The interventricular septum depolarizes normally when there is right bundle branch block. Accordingly, an abnormal Q wave due to myocardial infarction can be recorded in a patient with right bundle branch block. Therefore, when such an abnormal initial 0.04 second QRS abnormality is recorded in a patient with right bundle branch block, the block is considered to be complicated.

Right bundle branch block is complicated when the mean QRS vector is directed more than +120° to the right and anteriorly, suggesting additional posterior-inferior division block, or anteriorly to the left or superiorly, suggesting additional left anterior-division block.

A primary S-T segment abnormality may be present. In such cases the S-T segment vector is not parallel with the mean T vector; the spatial angle between the S-T and T vectors may be greater than 60° (5).

A primary T wave abnormality may be present. Such an abnormality is identified by constructing the ventricular gradient; the gradient is abnormal when there is a primary T wave abnormality.

An example of right bundle branch block complicated by primary S-T segment abnormality and a primary T wave abnormality is depicted in Figure 16-8.

Complicated Right Bundle Branch Block
Plus Left Anterior-Superior Division
Block

Complicated right bundle branch block plus left anterior-superior division block is believed to be present when the following electrocardiographic abnormalities are present.

The duration of the QRS complex is 0.12 second or greater.

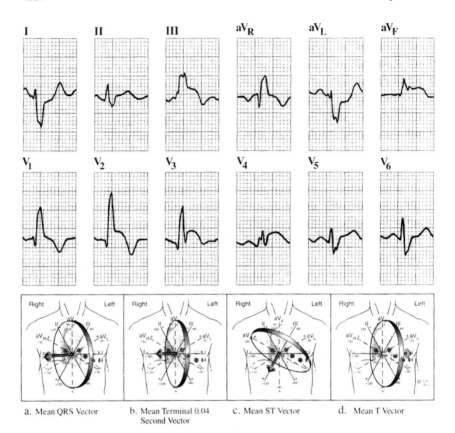

a. Mean QRS Vector   b. Mean Terminal 0.04   c. Mean ST Vector   d. Mean T Vector
                         Second Vector

Figure 16-8 This electrocardiogram, showing complicated right bundle branch block due to possible left posterior-inferior division block and inferoanterior epicardial injury, was recorded from a 56-year-old man with an acute myocardial infarction. The P waves are normal and the P-R interval is 0.15 second. The duration of the QRS complexes is 0.12 to 0.13 second. In *a*, the mean QRS vector is directed at +175° in the frontal plane and about 45° to 50° anteriorly. This degree of rightward deviation of the mean QRS vector is more than is seen in usual tracing showing right bundle branch block. In *b*, the mean terminal 0.04 second QRS vector is directed at ±180° in the frontal plane and about 20° to 30° anteriorly. In *c*, the large mean S-T vector is directed at +120° in the frontal plane and 30° anteriorly. The S-T—T angle is larger than 60° and this indicates a

The direction of the initial 0.01 to 0.02 QRS second vector may be normal because the depolarization of the septum is altered very little. An abnormal Q wave due to an altered direction of the first 0.02 to 0.04 second of the QRS complex can develop secondary to myocardial infarction.

The mean QRS vector is directed anteriorly but is directed more than −30° to the left or superiorly. This

---

definite primary S-T wave abnormality. The mean T vector is directed at 0° in the frontal plane and 35° posteriorly. The ventricular gradient is abnormal, indicating a primary T wave abnormality. This interesting tracing showing complicated right bundle branch block and inferoanterior myocardial infarction illustrates several points.

The mean QRS vector is directed more than +120° to the right, which is usually not seen in uncomplicated right bundle branch block. This could be due to associated left posterior-inferior division block or infarctions of the lateral wall of the left ventricle.

The mean S-T segment vector is directed at +120° in the frontal plane and anteriorly. The direction of the S-T vector should lead the interpreter to consider the extension of the inferior infarct to include the right ventricle or extensive inferoanterior infarction, including infarction of the septum.

A coronary arteriogram in this patient revealed 80% diameter obstruction of the left anterior descending coronary artery, which wrapped around the cardiac apex, 70% obstruction of the first diagonal and only 60% obstruction of the right coronary artery. These findings support the view that this particular tracing is the result of extensive inferior-anterior and septal infarction of the left ventricle. (*Source*: Hurst JW. *Cardiovascular Diagnosis: The Initial Examination*. St. Louis: Mosby-Year Book, Inc, 1993:344. The author, J.W.H., owns the copyright.)

unusual direction of the mean QRS vector should be
detected immediately.

The terminal 0.04 second QRS vector is directed anteriorly, but is directed far to the left or superiorly as
much as $-60°$ to $-120°$ in the frontal plane. Remember, in the abnormality being discussed here, the left
anterior-superior division branch of the left ventricular conduction system is blocked in addition to the
right bundle. Therefore, the unusual direction of the
terminal 0.04 second QRS vector is due to the summation of two opposing electrical forces. Accordingly,
the abnormal terminal portion of the QRS complex
is produced by the late depolarization of the left ventricle, facilitated by an intact left posterior-inferior
division, causing the terminal QRS forces to be directed to the left and superiorly from $-60°$ to $-120°$,
plus the late abnormal depolarization of the right
ventricle, facilitated by the right bundle branch
block, causing the terminal QRS forces to be directed
anteriorly.

Complicated right bundle branch block plus left anterior-
superior division block can be caused by coronary atherosclerotic heart disease with multiple infarctions, cardiomyopathy,
an ostium primum atrial septal defect, primary disease of the
conduction system, certain drugs, and cardiac surgery.

Two electrocardiograms of complicated right bundle
branch block plus left anterior-superior division block are
shown in Figures 16-9 and 16-10.

Complicated Right Bundle Branch Block
Plus Left Posterior-Inferior Division
Block

This abnormality of the conduction system of the ventricles is
the most difficult conduction defect to establish with certainty.
The condition is believed to be present when the following electrocardiographic abnormalities are present.

The duration of the QRS complex is 0.12 second or more. The measurement should be made by viewing the QRS complexes rather than accepting the computer readout.

Initial 0.01 to 0.02 second QRS vector may be directed normally unless an abnormal Q wave vector is present.

The mean QRS vector is directed +120° or more to the right and anteriorly. The mean QRS vector that characterizes uncomplicated right bundle branch block is usually directed less than +120° to the right. Herein lies the problem of identifying right bundle branch block plus left posterior-inferior division block—other mechanisms may be responsible for the shift of the mean QRS vector beyond +120°. For example, the electrocardiogram of patients with right ventricular dilatation may exhibit right bundle branch block and the mean QRS vector is commonly directed more than 120° to the right. My colleagues and I reported on a group of patients who had total correction of tetralogy of Fallot early in life and found that almost all of those patients whose QRS duration was more than 0.14 second, and in whom the mean QRS vector was directed toward the northwest quadrant of the hexaxial references system, had dilated right ventricles and right ventricular dysfunction proved with MRI studies (4). It is therefore necessary to exclude the presence of right ventricular dilatation, or the clinical setting where such could be possible, before concluding that the cause of a mean QRS vector directed more than 120° to the right is due to a block in the left posterior-inferior division of the left ventricular conduction system.

The terminal 0.04 second QRS vector is directed far to the right and anteriorly. It is a summation vector produced by the electrical forces created by right bundle branch block plus by the electrical forces pro-

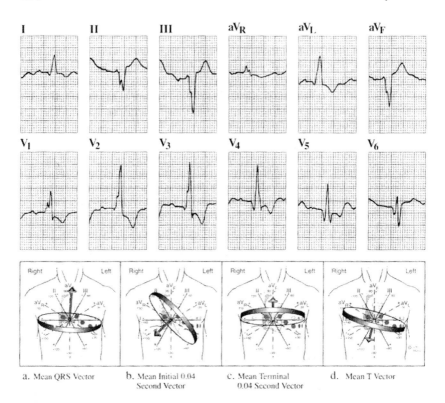

I II III aV$_R$ aV$_L$ aV$_F$

V$_1$ V$_2$ V$_3$ V$_4$ V$_5$ V$_6$

a. Mean QRS Vector   b. Mean Initial 0.04   c. Mean Terminal   d. Mean T Vector
                          Second Vector   0.04 Second Vector

Figure 16-9 This electrocardiogram, showing complicated right bundle branch block plus left anterior-superior division block, was recorded from a 69-year-old man with a lateral myocardial infarction. The P waves are not seen clearly in the extremity leads, but the P-R interval is 0.23 second. The duration of the QRS complexes is 0.16 second. In *a*, the mean QRS vector is directed at about −85° in the frontal plane and 20°–30° anteriorly. This produces negative QRS deflections in leads II and III and positive QRS deflection in leads V$_1$ through V$_4$. The mean initial 0.04 second QRS vector is directed at +140° in the frontal plane and about 20° anteriorly. This abnormality is the result of a lateral endocardial dead zone. The mean terminal 0.04 second QRS vector is directed at −90° in the frontal plane and 10° posteriorly. The unusual direction of the terminal mean 0.04 second QRS vector is because it is the vector sum of the electrical forces produced by the myocytes stimulated by the right

duced by the anterior portions of the left ventricle because the left posterior-inferior division of the left
conduction system is blocked.

When the mean S-T vector is directed within 30° to 60°
of the mean T vector, it is considered to be a secondary S-T segment displacement and is the result of
the repolarization process. A large S-T vector directed more than 60° away from the mean T vector
may be a primary S-T segment vector caused by epicardial injury of infarction.

The mean T vector is directed 120° to 180° away from the
mean QRS vector. When the ventricular gradient is
normal, the T vector is considered to be a secondary
T wave abnormality. When the ventricular gradient
is abnormal, there is a primary T wave abnormality,
which implies that a primary cause for an epicardial
alteration of repolarization is present.

When a recent previous tracing reveals no conduction abnormalities or evidence of right ventricular hypertrophy and
the new tracing shows complicated right bundle branch block
with the mean QRS vector directed more than 120° to the

---

bundle and the left anterior-superior division bundle. In most cases
it is directed more anteriorly than it is in this illustration but in this
case, it appears that there were more posterior forces influencing
the electrical field than there were anterior forces. In *d*, the mean
T vector is directed at +100° in the frontal plane and 20° posteriorly.
The ventricular gradient is abnormal, signifying a primary T wave
abnormality.

There are several different causes for this type of conduction
defect, including atherosclerotic coronary heart disease, cardiomyopathy, ostium primum, and primary disease of the conduction system. The abnormal Q waves in this patient favor the diagnosis of
myocardial infarction. (*Source*: Hurst JW. *Cardiovascular Diagnosis. The Initial Examination*. St. Louis: Mosby-Year Book, Inc, 1993:
354. The author, J.W.H., owns the copyright.)

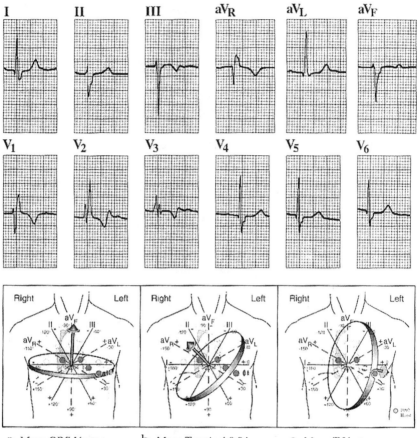

a. Mean QRS Vector   b. Mean Terminal 0.04   c. Mean T Vector
                               Second Vector

Figure 16-10 This electrocardiogram, showing right bundle branch block plus left anterior-superior division block, was recorded from a 17-year-old adolescent with an ostium primum atrial septal defect. The P waves are not shown in all leads but can be seen in leads I, aV_L, and V_4. The P-R interval is 0.21 second. The duration of the QRS complexes is 0.12 second. In *a*, the mean QRS vector is directed at $-85°$ in the frontal plane and about 30° anteriorly. This produces negative QRS complexes in leads II and III and positive QRS complexes in leads V_1 through V_4. In *b*, the mean terminal 0.04 second QRS vector is directed at about $-135°$ in the frontal plane

right, it is acceptable to consider the presence of additional left posterior-inferior division block. A patient with such a tracing could have myocardial infarction, myocarditis, or cardiomyopathy.

When there is no previous tracing available, but the patient exhibits the clinical picture of myocardial infarction with right bundle branch block in which the mean QRS vector is directed more than +120° to the right, it is customary to blame the findings on a conduction abnormality in the right bundle plus a defect in the left posterior-inferior division branch of the left ventricular conduction system. Even in this circumstance, right ventricular dilatation must be excluded, and infarction of the lateral wall of the left ventricle could cause the marked shift of the mean QRS vector to the right.

An electrocardiogram showing complicated right bundle branch block plus possible left posterior-inferior division block is shown in Figure 16-8.

NONDESCRIPT VENTRICULAR CONDUCTION SYSTEM ABNORMALITIES

The commonly observed ventricular conduction system defects were described in the previous pages of this chapter. There

---

and 40° anteriorly. In *c*, the mean T vector is directed at +10° in the frontal plane and about 40° posteriorly. The T wave is abnormal for the QRS because the ventricular gradient is abnormal. This electrocardiogram shows complicated right bundle branch block plus left anterior-superior division block. Such a tracing may be seen in patients with coronary atherosclerotic heart disease, cardiomyopathy, ostium primum atrial septal defect, primary disease of the conduction system (Lenegre disease), or Lev disease. This electrocardiogram was recorded from a patient with an ostium primum atrial septal defect. (*Source*: Hurst JW. *Cardiovascular Diagnosis. The Initial Examination*. St. Louis: Mosby-Year Book, Inc, 1993:338. The author, J.W.H., owns the copyright.)

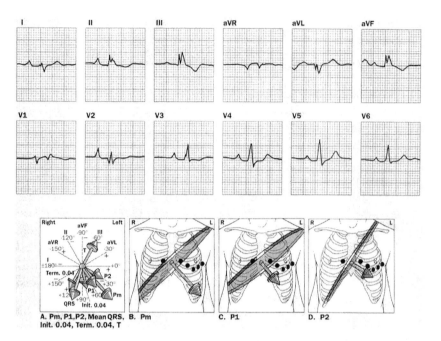

| I | II | III | aVR | aVL | aVF |

| V1 | V2 | V3 | V4 | V5 | V6 |

A. Pm, P1,P2, Mean QRS, B. Pm   C. P1   D. P2
Init. 0.04, Term. 0.04, T

Figure 16-11   This electrocardiogram, showing abnormal P waves, abnormal initial mean 0.04 second QRS forces, abnormal terminal mean 0.04 second QRS forces, and low QRS amplitude, was recorded from a 36-year-old woman with Ebstein anomaly of the tricuspid valve. The P waves are abnormal and the P-R interval is 0.22 second. The QRS duration is 0.13 second. The diagnostic vectors are shown in *a*. In *b*, the mean P vector (P_m) is large. It is directed at +45° in the frontal plane and anterior or parallel with the frontal plane. Right atrial depolarization (P_1) and left atrial depolarization (P_2) are directed similarly, with P_1 being directed only a few degrees anterior to P_2. Note the size of the P wave in lead V_2 where it measures more than 2.5 millimeters high. Note also that the P wave is pointed and that the second half of the P wave measures more than -0.04 millimeter second in lead V_1. This is usually due to left atrial depolarization, but when the right atrium is huge, the second half of the P wave may be negative in lead V_1 because the depolarization process turns posteriorly in the huge right atrium on its way to the left atrium. The QRS complexes exhibit less amplitude in this tracing than is usually seen in patients with QRS conduction defects. The

are, however, many examples of conduction abnormalities that do not fit into such a classification. Some of these nondescript abnormalities are probably caused by the vector sum of several abnormalities of the terminal depolarization process.

Here are some of the features of nondescript ventricular conduction abnormalities.

> The duration of the QRS complexes may be 0.16 to 0.20 second. This suggests a large heart with damage to the entire conduction system. It may be caused by dilated cardiomyopathy from any cause, certain drugs, hyperkalemia, or hypothermia.
>
> Conditions such as "peri-infarction" block can produce QRS terminal force abnormalities that do not fit the attributes of the usual conduction abnormalities.
>
> Ordinarily, the QRS *amplitude* increases when the QRS

---

mean QRS vector is directed at +110° in the frontal plane and is parallel with the frontal plane. The mean initial 0.04 second QRS second vector is directed at +80° in the frontal plane and slightly posterior. The initial forces are directed more posteriorly than the subsequent QRS forces. The mean terminal 0.04 second QRS vector is directed at +120° in the frontal plane and is parallel with the frontal plane. The mean T vector is directed at −60° in the frontal plane and about 20° posteriorly. The direction of the ventricular gradient is directed at about +15°. This is an unusual tracing. There is a right atrial abnormality. The second half of the P wave is negative in lead V_1, suggesting a left atrial abnormality. Note, however, that it is pointed, suggesting that there is a right atrial abnormality (see text). There is some type of right ventricular conduction defect, but the amplitude of the terminal QRS forces is much less than is usually seen. This abnormality can be explained by realizing that patients with Ebstein anomaly have small right ventricles. The abnormal P waves and abnormal QRS complexes in this tracing are characteristic of Ebstein anomaly of the heart. (*Source:* Hurst JW. *Ventricular Electrocardiography.* New York: Gower Medical Publishing, 1991:7.3. The author, J.W.H., owns the copyright.)

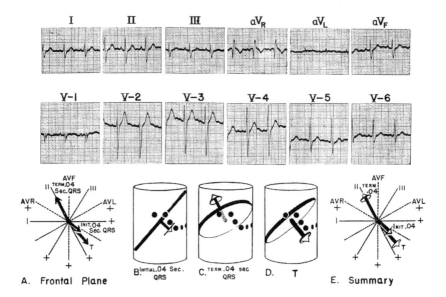

Figure 16-12 This electrocardiogram, showing the S_1, S_2, S_3 type of conduction defect, was recorded from a 24-year-old normal subject. The P waves are normal and the P-R interval is 0.14 second. The duration of the QRS complexes is 0.08 second. The mean QRS vector is difficult to compute because the QRS complexes are equaphasic in the extremity leads. The mean QRS vector is probably directed at about $-105°$ in the frontal plane and slightly posterior. In a, b, and c, the initial mean 0.04 second QRS vector is directed at $+50°$ in the frontal plane and is parallel with the frontal plane. The mean terminal 0.04 second QRS vector is directed at $-120°$ in the frontal plane and moderately posterior. The mean T vector is directed at about $+50°$ in the frontal plane and about $5°$ to $10°$ anteriorly. This type of conduction defect may occur in otherwise normal hearts. It is believed by some investigators to be caused by an alteration of the Purkinje fibers in the right ventricle. The abnormality may also occur in patients with obstructive pulmonary disease or hypertrophic cardiomyopathy. (*Source*: Hurst JW, Woodson GC Jr: *Atlas of Spatial Vector Electrocardiography*. New York: The Blakiston Company, Inc, 1951:169. The author, J.W.H., owns the copyright.)

complexes widens. This is thought to occur because electrical forces are no longer located diametrically opposite each other and do not cancel each other out. The QRS amplitude is *decreased* in some patients with a QRS duration of 0.14 to 0.16 second. Does this imply that nonviable myocytes are unable to contribute to the depolarization process?

Some patients with complex congenital heart diseases exhibit bizarre ventricular conduction defects. This is probably caused by anomalies of the conduction system itself plus abnormalities of the ventricular muscle. For example, the electrocardiogram of a patient with Ebstein's anomaly is interesting because complicated right bundle branch block may be present but the terminal 0.04 second QRS vector is not large, because the right ventricle is small (see Fig. 16-11).

The S_1, S_2, S_3 conduction defect is an unusual defect characterized by a normal QRS duration and a terminal 0.04 second QRS vector that is directed superiorly. This vector is about equal in amplitude to the initial 0.04 second QRS vector that is directed normally. This conduction defect may occur in subjects that have no other discernible heart disease, in patients with obstructive pulmonary disease (6), and in patients with hypertrophic cardiomyopathy. An electrocardiogram showing an S_1, S_2, S_3 conduction defect is depicted in Figure 16-12.

REFERENCES

1. Tawara S. *Das reizleitungssystem des saugetierherzens.* Jena, Gustav Fischer, 1906.

2. Laiken N, Laiken SL, Karliner JS. *Interpretation of Electrocardiograms: A self-instructional approach*, 2nd ed. New York: Raven Press, 1988:100–103.

3. Laiken N, Laiken SL, Karliner JS. *Interpretation of Electrocar-*

diograms: A self-instructional approach, 2nd ed. New York: Raven Press, 1988:104–107.

4. Book WM, Parks WJ, Hopkins KL, Hurst JW. Electrocardiographic predictors of right ventricular volume measured by magnetic resonance imaging late after total repair of Tetralogy of Fallot. Clin Cardiol 1999;22:740–746.

5. Hurst JW. Abnormalities of the S-T segment—Part I & II. Clin Cardiol 1997;20:511–520, 595–600.

6. de Luna AB, Carrió I, Subirana MT, Torner P, Cosín J, Sagués F, Guindo J. Electrophysiological mechanisms of the S_I S_{II} S_{III} electrocardiographic morphology. J Electrocardiology 1987; 20(1):38–44.

Chapter 17

The Electrocardiographic Signs of Pericarditis

Pericarditis is usually generalized, but occasionally it is localized (1). The pericardium produces no electrical forces, but the condition produces epicardial damage that is responsible for the electrocardiographic abnormalities.

THE ELECTROCARDIOGRAPHIC SIGNS OF ACUTE GENERALIZED PERICARDITIS

Atrial fibrillation may occasionally develop.

The P-Q segment may be displaced downward. This abnormality may not be seen in all leads, so a mean vector cannot be visualized.

The amplitude of the QRS complex may be decreased if there is *pericardial fluid*. The 12-lead total QRS amplitude will be on the low side of the normal range, which is 80 to 185 millimeters. When pericardial fluid is present there may be *electrical alternans* of the QRS complexes. This is because of a "swinging heart" that produces a different electrical field every other beat.

The initial 0.04 second QRS vector remains normally directed.

The mean S-T segment vector is directed toward the centroid of an infinite number of electrical forces that are directed toward the epicardial surface of the entire heart. Accordingly, this produces a mean S-T vector that is almost parallel with the anatomic axis of the heart and is directed toward the cardiac apex. This usually produces elevation of the S-T segments in the extremity leads I, II, III, aV_F, and in leads V_3-V_6. The mean S-T vector in such cases is directed at about $+30°$ to $+60°$ in the frontal plane and is almost parallel with the frontal plane. Accordingly, the S-T segment when represented as a vector may be slightly depressed, slightly elevated, or isoelectric in lead aV_L and displaced downward in lead aV_R.

The mean T vector may initially be directed normally, but as the S-T vector diminishes, the mean T vector may be directed opposite the cardiac apex, producing an inverted T waves in leads I, II, III, aV_F, and possibly aV_L and in leads V_4-V_6.

As time passes, the S-T segment vector becomes smaller and the mean T vector becomes larger. Later still, the T wave abnormality may disappear or a small T wave abnormality may persist.

Pericarditis due to viral infection is generalized. The pericarditis due to uremia is generalized but it does not produce epicardial damage as described with infective pericarditis. A

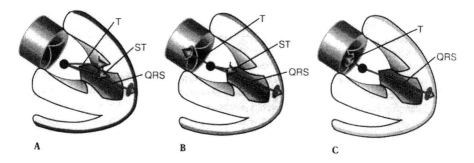

Figure 17-1 Electrocardiographic abnormalities produced by acute pericarditis. *A.* Pericarditis usually produces generalized epicardial myocardial injury (see dark area). Initially, during the early stage of pericarditis, an arrow representing the mean of the electrical forces (vectors) responsible for the ST segment is directed toward the anatomic apex of the left ventricle. It is produced by generalized epicardial injury. The PQ segment may become displaced downward in leads where the P waves are upright. It cannot be represented by an arrow, because it is rarely seen in all leads. *B.* During the second stage of acute pericarditis, the arrow representing the ST segment vector becomes smaller than it was in *A*, and an arrow representing the mean of the electrical forces (vectors) responsible for the T wave is directed somewhat opposite to the anatomic apex of the left ventricle; it is due to generalized epicardial iischemia. *C.* During the third stage of acute pericarditis an arrow representing the mean of the electrical forces (vectors) responsible for the ST segment decreases markedly, and the arrow representing the mean of the electrical forces (vectors) responsible for the T wave may become larger than it was in *B*. The T waves may then decrease in size, as shown here. When pericardial fluid develops, the amplitude of the QRS complexes and T waves decreases, and electrical alternans of the QRS complexes and T waves may appear. (*Source*: Hurst JW. *Cardiovascular Diagnosis. The Initial Examination.* St. Louis: Mosby-Year Book, Inc, 1993:392. The author, J.W.H., owns the copyright.)

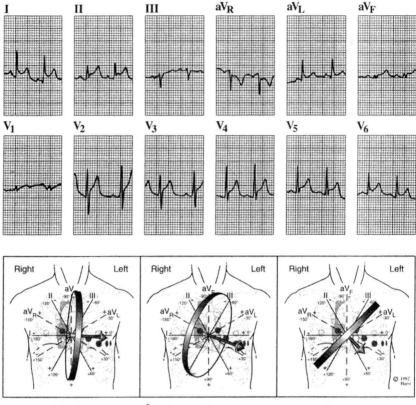

a. Mean QRS Vector   b. Mean ST Vector   c. Mean T Vector

Figure 17-2 This electrocardiogram was recorded from a 68-year-old man with acute pericarditis associated with rheumatoid arthritis. The P waves are normal and the P-R interval is 0.14 second. The duration of the QRS complexes is 0.08 second and the QT interval is 0.28 second. The P-Q segment is displaced downward in leads I and II. In *a*, the mean QRS vector is directed at +5° in the frontal plane and about 5° posteriorly. The amplitude of the QRS complexes is normal. In *b*, the mean S-T vector is directed at about +20° in the frontal plane and 20° to 30° anteriorly, indicating generalized epicardial injury. In *c*, the mean T vector is directed at +45° in the frontal plane and is parallel with the frontal plane. The displaced P-Q segment and the S-T vector due to generalized epicardial injury are major clues that the abnormalities are caused by generalized pericarditis. (*Source:* Hurst JW. *Cardiovascular Diagnosis. The Initial Examination.* St. Louis: Mosby-Year Book, Inc, 1993:394. The author, J.W.H., owns the copyright.)

loud pericardial rub may be heard in uremic patients but the electrocardiographic signs of pericarditis do not develop; the electrocardiographic abnoramlities are commonly caused by electrolyte abnormalities in such patients (2). Spodick, an expert in pericarditis, believes that an electrocardiogram recorded from a uremic patient showing the abnormalities of pericarditis suggests that the patient has viral pericarditis rather than uremic pericarditis (2).

The S-T and T wave abnormalities of apical myocardial infarction may simulate those of pericarditis. As discussed in Chapter 15, abnormal Q waves may not develop in patients with apical infarction, because the aortic and mitral valves are opposite the cardiac apex rather than intact myocardium that is needed to produce an abnormal Q wave. When the S-T vector is huge in such cases it suggests infarction, but this is not a reliable sign, because the S-T segment displacement is not huge in all patients with infarction.

The various electrocardiographic stages of pericarditis are illustrated in Figure 17-1. The electrocardiogram of a patient with acute pericarditis is shown in Figure 17-2. An electrocardiogram showing electrical alternans due to pericardial fluid is shown in Figure 17-3.

LOCALIZED PERICARDITIS

Pericarditis may be localized and segmental. For example, localized pericarditis may occur with myocardial infarction. When it does, the S-T segment vector that initially represented epicardial injury due to the infarction may become larger. In general, one can conclude that the appearance of segmental or localized pericarditis depends on a localizing factor, such as infarction, the surgeon's knife, or neoplastic disease (especially of the lung).

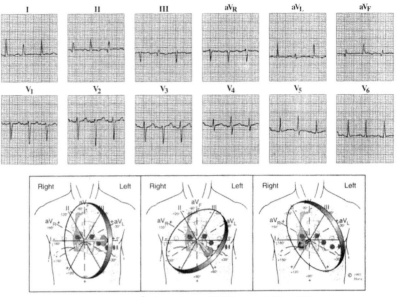

a. First Mean QRS Vector   b. Second Mean QRS Vector   c. Mean T Vector

Figure 17-3   This electrocardiogram was recorded from a 40-year-old man with pericardial effusion due to involvement of the pericardium with sarcoma of the thymus. The P waves are normal. The duration of the QRS complexes is 0.08 second. The Q-T interval is 0.28 second. The amplitude of the QRS complexes is 90 to 100 millimeters. Ths is on the low end of the normal 12-lead QRS amplitude (normal range is 80 to 185 millimeters). Note the amplitude of the QRS complexes alternate in size every other complex. *This is called electrical alternans.* The mean T vector is directed at about +150° to the right 85° to 90° anteriorly. This tracing is diagnostic of pericarditis with pericardial effusion. (*Source*: Hurst JW. *Cardiovascular Diagnosis. The Initial Examination*. St. Louis: Mosby-Year Book, Inc, 1993:396. The author, J.W.H., owns the copyright.)

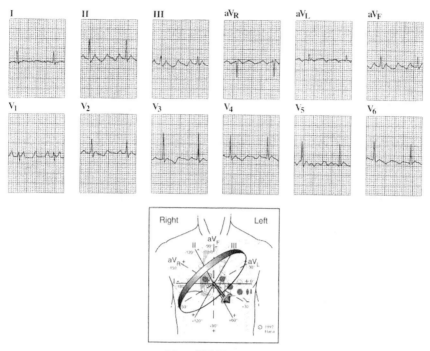

Mean QRS Vector

Figure 17-4 This electrocardiogram was recorded from a 24-year-old woman with calcific constrictive pericarditis. Atrial flutter is present with 3:1 atriventricular block. The ventricular rate is about 77. The duration of the QRS complexes is 0.08 second. The mean QRS vector is directed at about +50° in the frontal plane and about 10° anteriorly. The 12-lead QRS amplitude is about 78 millimeters (80 to 185 millimeters is the normal range). The atrial flutter and low QRS amplitude suggest pericardial disease. The abnormalities could also occur in patients with dilated or restrictive cardiomyopathy. (*Source*: Hurst JW. *Cardiovascular Diagnosis. The Initial Examination*. St. Louis: Mosby-Year Book, Inc, 1993:398. The author, J.W.H., owns the copyright. Electrocardiogram courtesy of Dr. Paul F. Walter, Emory University Hospital, Atlanta, Georgia.)

THE ELECTROCARDIOGRAM ASSOCIATED
WITH CONSTRICTIVE PERICARDITIS

Constrictive pericarditis may produce atrial fibrillation, low
QRS amplitude, and an abnormal mean T vector (see Fig.
17-4).

THE ELECTROCARDIOGRAPHIC SIGNS
OF MYOPERICARDITIS

Severe myocarditis and pericarditis may appear in the same
patient and this condition is called myopericarditis. The electrocardiogram may show the S-T and T wave changes of pericarditis and the QRS complex may show abnormal initial QRS
forces imitating the abnormal Q waves of myocardial infarction (see Chapter 15). The following point is germane to
the subject: an abnormality of the initial 0.03 to 0.04 second
of the QRS complex may produce Q waves in leads where no
Q waves should be present. Such abnormalities are commonly
caused by myocardial infarction due to coronary atherosclerotic heart disease. The basic problem, however, is that myocytes that are destroyed by other diseases, such as myocarditis
or infiltration diseases of the myocardium, can produce a similar effect. It is wise to remember all the conditions that may
alter the initial portion of the QRS complex when the electrocardiogram is interpreted.

REFERENCES

1. Spodick DH. *The Pericardium: A Comprehensive Textbook*. New
   York: Marcel Dekker, 1997;1–464.

2. Spodick DH. *The Pericardium: A Comprehensive Textbook*. New
   York: Marcel Dekker, 1997:293.

Chapter 18

Electrocardiographic Abnormalities Due to Pulmonary Embolism

Pulmonary embolism is a sneaky disease and continues to be a common and unexpected cause of acute pulmonary disease and death.

THE ELECTROCARDIOGRAPHIC ABNORMALITIES PRODUCED BY ACUTE PULMONARY EMBOLISM (1)

A small pulmonary embolism may not produce any abnormalities in the electrocardiogram.

Sinus tachycardia may be present. A large pulmonary embolism may precipitate junctional supraventricular tachycardia or atrial fibrillation.

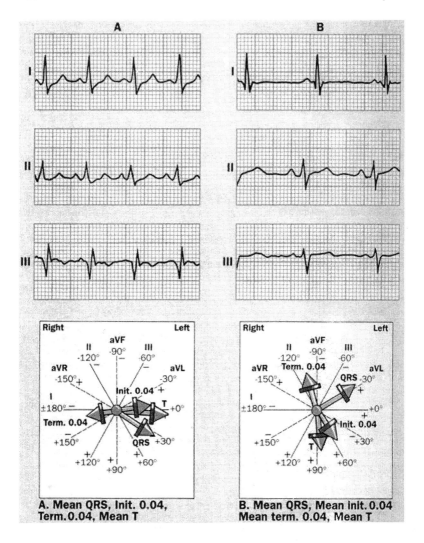

A. Mean QRS, Init. 0.04,
Term. 0.04, Mean T

B. Mean QRS, Mean Init. 0.04
Mean term. 0.04, Mean T

Figure 18-1 This electrocardiogram shows the electrocardiographic abnormalities described by McGinn and White (2). *A.* The initial mean 0.04 second QRS vector is shifted to the left producing a large Q wave in lead III. The mean terminal 0.04 second QRS vector is directed to the right, producing a large S wave in lead I. The mean T vector is directed to the left. This electrocardiogram was recorded 2 hours after acute pulmonary embolism. *B.* This tracing

The duration of the QRS complexes may remain normal or increase in duration; right ventricular conduction delay or right bundle branch block may develop acutely.

A large pulmonary embolism produces acute hypoxia and causes acute dilatation of the right ventricle. This may cause a shift in the position of the interventricular septum. This alters the direction of the initial QRS vector so that initial QRS forces become directed to the left. The new direction of the initial QRS forces may imitate inferior myocardial infarction. The acute dilatation of the right ventricle also produces right ventricular conduction delay so that the terminal portion of the QRS complexes may be directed to the right and anteriorly, producing new S waves in leads I, and V_6 and an R prime wave in lead V_1. This has been referred to as the McGinn-White syndrome (see Fig. 18-1) (2).

The mean S-T vector may be directed to the right and superiorly, indicating subendocardial injury. This is most likely due to severe myocardial ischemia associated with hypoxia.

The mean T vector may be directed to the left and posteriorly away from the right ventricle. This abnormality may be erroneously attributed to anterior myocardial infarction (see Fig. 18-2).

---

was recorded 4 weeks after the tracing shown in A. It reveals the disappearance of the abnormalities shown in A. The tracing is abnormal, but the signs of pulmonary embolism are no longer present. (*Source*: Top: McGinn S, White PD. Acute cor pulmonale resulting from pulmonary embolism: Its clinical recognition. *JAMA* 1935; 104(17): 1475. Used with permission. Bottom: Hurst JW. *Ventricular Electrocardiography*. New York: Gower Medical Publishing 1991: 13.10. The author, J.W.H., owns the copyright.)

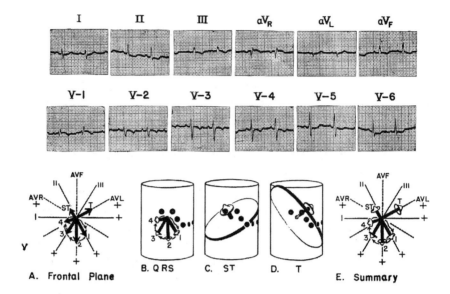

Figure 18-2 This electrocardiogram, showing the abnormalities caused by acute pulmonary embolism, was recorded shortly after a 54-year-old man experienced severe dyspnea. In *a* and *b*, the initial spatial QRS forces in this patient are directed normally. The terminal spatial QRS forces are directed to the right and anteriorly indicating right ventricular conduction delay. This finding, when observed in the appropriate clinical setting, should suggest acute pulmonary embolism. In *c*, the mean S-T segment vector is directed at −120° in the frontal plane and about 70° anteriorly, suggesting endocardial injury. In *d*, the mean T vector is directed at −20° in the frontal plane and about 50° posteriorly, sugesting an abnormality of the repolarization process anteriorly; in this patient the anterior repolarization abnormality is in the right ventricle. The abnormalities shown in this electrocardiogram were caused by an acute pulmonary embolism. However, most pulmonary emboli do not produce all of these abnormalities. (*Source*: Hurst JW, Woodson GC Jr: *Atlas of Spatial Vector Electrocardiography*. New York: The Blakiston Company, Inc, 1951:203. The author, J.W.H., owns the copyright.)

The electrocardiographic signs of right ventricular hypertrophy due to systolic pressure overload of the right ventricle may develop in patients with repeated pulmonary emboli (see Chapter 14).

REFERENCES

1. Stein PD, Dalen JE, McIntyre KM, Sasahara AA, Wenger NK, Willis PW III. The electrocardiogram in acute pulmonary embolism. Prog Cardiovasc Dis 1975;27(4):247.

2. McGinn S, White PD. Acute cor pulmonale resulting from pulmonary embolism: Its clinical recognition. JAMA 1935;104(17): 1475.

Chapter 19

Electrocardiographic Abnormalities Due to Chronic Obstructive Lung Disease with Emphysema

The electrocardiographic abnormalities produced by chronic obstructive pulmonary disease with emphysema include the following:

Sinus tachycardia and atrial fibrillation may develop.
Patients with normal rhythm may exhibit electrocardiographic signs of right atrial abnormality. The direction of the mean P vector is commonly directed at +70° or more in the frontal plane. This is thought by Spodick and his coworkers to be due to the change in the heart's position because the diaphragm is located lower in the chest in patients with emphysema than it is normally (1).

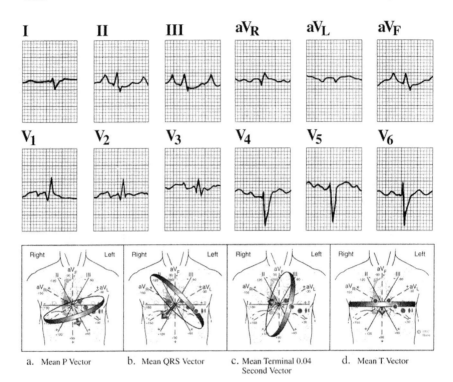

a. Mean P Vector   b. Mean QRS Vector   c. Mean Terminal 0.04   d. Mean T Vector
                                                          Second Vector

Figure 19-1 This electrocardiogram shows the abnormalities caused by chronic obstructive lung disease due to pulmonary emphysema. In a, the mean P vector is directed at about $+70°$ in the frontal plane. The P wave is peaked and measures 2.5 millimeters high in lead II, suggesting right atrial abnormality. Although the second half of the P wave is negative in lead V_1, it does not measure -0.04 millimeter second. In b, the mean QRS vector is directed at $+135°$ in the frontal plane and about $20°$ anteriorly. The duration of the QRS complexes is about 0.12 second and the 12-lead QRS amplitude is 84 millimeters, which is on the low side of the normal range. In c, the mean terminal 0.04 second QRS vector is directed to the right and anteriorly. In d, the mean T vector is directed at $+90°$ in the frontal plane and is parallel with the frontal plane. The right atrial abnormality, consisting of a taller-than-average P wave and a mean P vector that is directed about $+70°$ to the right, the right bundle

The amplitude of the QRS complexes and T waves may be diminished when there is pulmonary emphysema.

Right ventricular conduction delay or right bundle branch block may develop. An S_1, S_2, S_3 conduction abnormality may appear.

The mean T vector may be directed to the left and posteriorly.

When the electrocardiographic abnormalities listed above develop in a patient with pulmonary emphysema, one can conclude that the lung disease is severe. Stated another way, considerable chronic obstructive pulmonary disease can be present and the electrocardiogram may remain normal.

An electrocardiogram from a patient with chronic obstructive lung disease and emphysema is shown in Figure 19-1.

REFERENCE

1. Baljepally R, Spodick DH. Electrocardiographic screening for emphysema: The frontal plane P axis. Clin Cardiol 1999;22:226–228.

---

branch block, and QRS amplitude that is on the low side of the normal range, suggest that the abnormalities are the result of chronic obstructive lung disease and emphysema. (*Source*: Top: The electrocardiogram is from Fowler NO, Daniels C, Scott RC, et al. The electrocardiogram in cor pulmonale with and without emphysema. *Am J Cardiol* 1965;16:501. Used with permission. Bottom: Hurst JW. *Cardiovascular Diagnosis. The Initial Examination.* St. Louis: Mosby-Year Book, Inc, 1993:400. The author, J.W.H., owns the copyright.)

Chapter 20

Effect of Digitalis on the Electrocardiogram

The ingestion of digitalis glycosides produces the following changes in the electrocardiogram (1).

> All types of rhythm disturbances can be produced by digitalis, including sinus bradycardia, sinus node Wenckebach, atrial arrhythmias, atrioventricular Wenckebach; all degrees of atrioventricular block; ventricular premature complexes; ventricular tachycardia; and ventricular fibrillation.
> Prolongation of the P-R interval may occur but this is less common than shortening of the Q-T interval.

The *duration* of the QRS complexes does not change in patients taking digitalis except when ventricular tachycardia develops.

The *direction and amplitude of the mean QRS vector and its components* are not altered by digitalis medication unless ventricular tachycardia develops.

The *direction* of a vector representing the last part of the T waves is not altered by digitalis; its *amplitude* is altered considerably so that it becomes shorter and shorter until it is barely visible.

As the last part of the T waves becomes smaller, *an S-T segment vector* develops. It is, in reality, the first part of the T wave but is traditionally referred to as an S-T segment. As the mean S-T vector becomes larger, the vector representing the last part of the T wave becomes smaller and the Q-T interval becomes shorter. The so-called mean S-T vector is directed almost opposite to the direction of the mean QRS vector.

The effect of digitalis medication is shown diagrammatically in Figure 20-1. Electrocardiograms showing the changes due to digitalis are shown in Figures 20-2 and 20-3.

The S-T and T wave abnormalities due to digitalis are the result of two physiological phenomena. Digitalis causes the repolarization process to occur earlier than usual; this shortens the Q-T interval. In addition, there appears to be a reversal of the repolarization process, suggesting that the normal transmyocardial pressure gradient is eliminated. The S-T segment abnormality is due to early repolarization of the ventricles. It is actually the early part of the T wave; it is not the result of a separate injury current.

It is interesting to note that digitalis effect may augment the electrical forces that are responsible for the S-T and T wave changes of ventricular hypertrophy. For example, the ingestion of digitalis may precipitate the S-T and T changes of

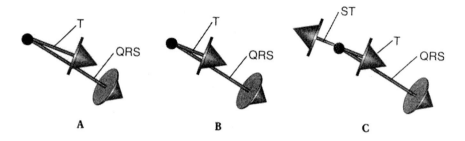

Figure 20-1 The effect of digitalis on the electrocardiogram. *A*. The normal direction of the mean QRS and mean T vectors in an adult prior to taking digitalis. The Q-T interval might be 0.38 second. *B*. The earliest effect of digitalis in the electrocardiogram. The direction of the mean QRS and mean T vectors remain the same as those shown in *A*. The mean T vector is smaller (shorter) than the mean T vector shown in A. The Q-T interval might be shorter than 0.38; it might be 0.34. *C*. A later stage of digitalis effect than was shown in *B*. Note the directions of the mean QRS vector and the vector representing the last part of the T waves have not changed. The vector representing the last part of the T waves has become even smaller (shorter) and a new S-T segment vector has developed. The mean S-T vector tends to be directed away from the direction of the mean QRS vector; it is actually the early part of the T wave. The Q-T interval might be even shorter than in A and B; it might be 0.32 second. (*Source*: Hurst JW. *Cardiovascular Diagnosis. The Initial Examination*. St. Louis: Mosby-Year Book, Inc, 1993:414. The author, J.W.H., owns the copyright.)

left ventricular hypertrophy in patients whose S-T and T wave vectors were previously normally directed.

The electrocardiographic signs of digitalis effect must be differentiated from the electrocardiographic abnormalities caused by the electrical current produced by endocardial injury. Endocardial injury is commonly produced by coronary atherosclerotic heart disease. In pure form, the abnormalities that are characteristic of endocardial injury include the following.

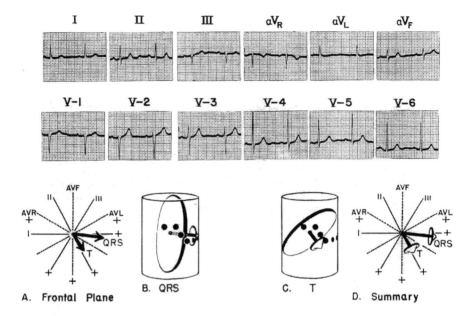

Figure 20-2 This electrocardiogram was recorded from a 77-year-old man with systemic hypertension. It was made prior to digitalis medication. The P waves are normal. The P-R interval is 0.16 second. The duration of the QRS complexes is 0.08 second. The Q-T interval is about 0.36 second. The mean QRS vector is directed at +10° in the frontal plane and about 30° posteriorly. The mean T vector is directed at +58° in the frontal plane and about 30° anteriorly. There is no S-T segment displacement. This electrocardiogram is normal although the QRS-T angle of 60° is borderline. (*Source*: Hurst JW, Woodson GC Jr. *Atlas of Spatial Vector Electrocardiography*. New York: The Blakiston Company, Inc, 1951:193. The author, J.W.H., owns the copyright.)

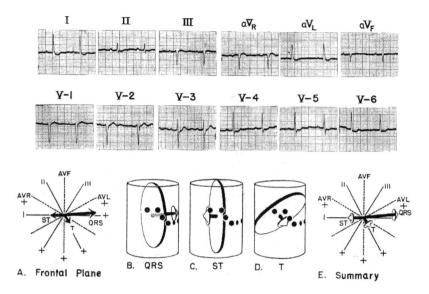

Figure 20-3 This electrocardiogram was made from the same patient whose tracing is shown in Figure 20-2, after taking digitalis. The P waves are normal. The P-R interval is 0.18 second. The duration of the QRS complexes is 0.08 second. The Q-T interval is difficult to measure, but is probably about 0.32 second (measured in lead V_2). The mean QRS vector is directed at $-10°$ in the frontal plane 30° posteriorly. The vector representing the last part of the T waves is small. It is probably directed at about $+58°$ in the frontal plane and about 30° anteriorly. The mean S-T vector is directed at $\pm180°$ in the frontal plane and about 20° to 30° anteriorly. It is actually the early part of the T waves. The abnormalities noted in this electrocardiogram are characteristic of the changes due to the ingestion of digitalis. (*Source*: Hurst JW, Woodson GC Jr. *Atlas of Spatial Vector Electrocardiography*. New York: The Blakiston Company, Inc, 1951: 195. The author, J.W.H., owns the copyright.)

The duration of the QRS complex and the direction of the mean QRS vector are unchanged from previous tracings in patients with endocardial injury.

The mean S-T vector is directed away from the cardiac apex, but the T waves and direction of the mean T vector remain unchanged from previous tracings. The T waves are likely to be normal or large. This is very different from the changes produced by digitalis when the last part of the T waves become smaller and smaller as the S-T segment displacement becomes larger.

The Q-T interval remains normal or may become longer than normal in patients with endocardial injury, whereas the Q-T internal is commonly decreased in duration in patients who are taking digitalis.

An electrocardiogram illustrating endocardial injury is shown in Figure 15-12.

Digitalis effect cannot always be separated from endocardial injury, and both abnormalities may be present in the same patient.

REFERENCE

1. Grant RP, Estes EH. *Spatial Vector Electrocardiography*. New York: The Blakiston Company, McGraw-Hill Book Co, 1951:90–95.

Chapter 21

Electrocardiographic Abnormalities Due to Hyperkalemia and Hypokalemia

ELECTROCARDIOGRAPHIC
ABNORMALITIES DUE TO HYPERKALEMIA

The Q-T interval may be prolonged.

The duration of the QRS complexes may be normal, but may be prolonged to 0.12 second or longer.

The direction of the mean QRS vector may become abnormal.

The direction of the terminal 0.04 second QRS vector may be altered. Various types of ventricular conduction abnormality may develop.

The shape, size, and duration of the T waves are altered. The T waves become large and peaked. The peaked

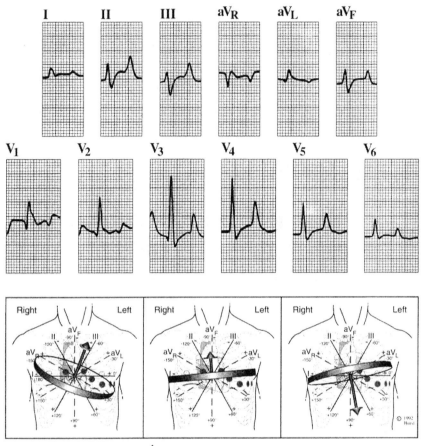

a. Mean QRS Vector   b. Mean Terminal 0.04   c. Mean T Vector
                             Second Vector

Figure 21-1 This electrocardiogram, showing abnormalities due to hyperkalemia, was recorded from an 85-year-old man with renal failure and diabetic acidosis. The serum potassium was 9.1 mEq/L. Junctional rhythm is present. The duration of the QRS complexes is 0.12 second. The Q-T interval is approximately 0.44 second. In *a*, the mean QRS vector is directed at about −70° in the frontal plane and at least 20° to 30° anteriorly. In *b*, the mean terminal 0.04 QRS vector is directed at about −95° in the frontal plane and parallel to the frontal plane. In *c*, the mean T vector is directed at about +80°

appearance is caused by the change in the ascending slope of the T waves in leads where the T waves are upright. Normally, the ascending slope of the T wave is more gradual than the downslope. Hyperkalemia causes the ascending and descending slopes of the T waves to be equally sloped; hence the term tent-shaped.

Hyperkalemia occurs in patients with renal failure. It is also seen in patients receiving potassium supplements, especially when they discontinue the potassium-losing diuretics given for heart failure but continue taking potassium supplements. There is a rough correlation of the abnormalities seen in the electrocardiogram with the serum level of potassium.

Normal T waves in patients with serum levels of potassium as high as 8 mEq/liter has been reported, but this is a rare exception to the general rule (1).

The hyperacute T waves of early myocardial infarction simulate the changes of hyperkalemia but the clinical setting is different (see Chapter 15).

The electrocardiographic signs of normal early repolarization may suggest hyperkalemia, but even though the T waves may be large, the ascending limb of the T wave is normally slanted and the clinical setting is different.

An electrocardiogram depicting the signs of hyperkalemia is shown in Figure 21-1.

---

in the frontal plane and about 10° anteriorly. The ventricular gradient is borderline normal. Note that the T waves are large, broad, and tent shaped. The abnormal rhythm, long Q-T interval, right bundle branch block plus left anterior-superior division block, broad-based tent-shaped T waves are characteristic of hyperkalemia. (*Source:* Hurst JW. *Cardiovascular Diagnosis. The Initial Examination.* St. Louis: Mosby-Year Book, Inc, 1993:412. The author, J.W.H., owns the copyright.)

ELECTROCARDIOGRAPHIC
ABNORMALITIES DUE TO HYPOKALEMIA

Atrial fibrillation may be present.

The duration of the QRS complexes is usually unchanged; it may be normal or abnormal.

The hallmark of the effect of hypokalemia on electrocardiograms is the development of large waves that were formerly called "U waves." These waves commonly join the T waves, producing what was formerly called a long Q-U interval.

According to Antzelevitch and his coworkers, the normal U wave is produced by repolarization of the His-Purkinje system (2–4). Such waves are never very large. Abnormally large or inverted U waves are not the result of this mechanism; they are caused by interrupted, or split, T waves. Antzelevitch has

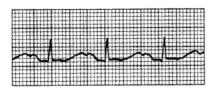

Figure 21-2 This short strip of an electrocardiogram, showing signs of hypokalemia and hypocalcemia, was recorded from a 57-year-old woman with cirrhosis of the liver. The serum potassium was 2.7 mEq/L and the serum calcium was 4.4 mg/%. The P-R interval is 0.21 second. The wave noted just before the P wave was formerly called a U wave. Such a wave is now thought to be the last part of an interrupted T wave. See text for a detailed explanation. The normal U wave is caused by repolarization of the His-Purkinje system, whereas an abnormal U wave is due to an interrupted T wave (2–4). So, what was formerly called a Q-U interval is, in reality, a Q-T interval. (*Source*: Hurst JW. *Cardiovascular Diagnosis. The Initial Examination*. St. Louis: Mosby-Year Book, Inc, 1993:410. The author, J.W.H., owns the copyright.)

proposed that these abnormal waves, which were formerly called U waves, are the result of an abnormality of repolarization of the ventricles. Normally the repolarization process produces one electrical gradient that passes from the epicardium to endocardium. Abnormal U waves are due to an interruption of the electrical gradient by the M cells that are located approximately in the mid-portion of the myocardium. The M cells look like other myocytes but are physiologically different in that their action potential lasts longer than it does in other myocytes. In addition, M cells react differently to catecholamine stimulation when compared to the reaction of other myo-

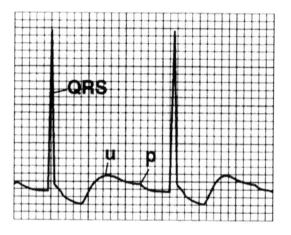

Figure 21-3   This electrocardiogram was recorded from a 33-year-old male with hypokalemic periodic paralysis. There was total paralysis of his arms and legs at the time of admission. His serum potassium at the time this electrocardiogram was recorded was 1.9 mEq/L. The electrocardiogram shows a prominent wave that was considered to be a large U wave. He gave a history of previous episodes, including one in which respiratory function was markedly diminished. Episodes were sometimes precipitated by large, high-carbohydate meals, such as the ingestion of pizza dough. (Tracing courtesy of Dr. David Propp, Emory University). (*Source*: Caplan LR, Hurst JW, Chimowitz MI. Clinical Neurocardiology. New York: Marcel Dekker 1999:390. Used with permission.)

cytes. When the M cells function abnormally, as they apparently do in patients with hypokalemia, they contribute to the development of two electrical gradients across the myocardium, causing an interrupted T wave. Accordingly, the abnormal U wave is now considered to be caused by the second portion of a split T wave.

Hypokalemia is caused by potassium-wasting diuretics, potassium-wasting diarrhea, and hypokalemic periodic paralysis.

Large or inverted U waves, or split T waves, may also be seen in the electrocardiograms of patients with hypertension, atherosclerotic heart disease, valve disease, and cardiomyopathy (5).

Electrocardiograms of patients showing the effect of low serum potassium are shown in Figures 21-2 and 21-3.

REFERENCES

1. Martinez-Vea A, Bardají A, Garcia C, Oliver JA. Severe hyperkalemia with minimal electrocardiographic manifestations: A report of seven cases. J Electrocardiol 1999;32:45–49.

2. Hurst JW. Naming of the waves in the ECG, with a brief account of their genesis. Circulation 1998;98:1937–1942.

3. Antzelevitch C. The M cell. J Cardiovasc Pharmacol Ther 1997; 2:73–76.

4. Antzelevitch C. November 26, 1999, personal communication.

5. Surawicz B. *Electrophysiologic basis of ECG and cardiac arrhythmias*. Baltimore: Williams & Wilkins, 1995:598–601.

Chapter 22

Electrocardiographic Abnormalities Due to Hypercalcemia and Hypocalcemia

THE ELECTROCARDIOGRAPHIC SIGNS OF HYPERCALCEMIA

Hypercalcemia shortens the S-T segment in the electrocardiogram. Unfortunately, it is difficult to determine when the S-T segment is abnormally short because there are no tables available that reveal the short side of the bell-shaped curve used to represent the normal range.

The direction of the mean S-T segment vector and mean T vector may suggest digitalis effect (see Fig. 22-1). It should be emphasized that digitalis should not be given to a patient with hypercalcemia, because the combination may produce ventricular fibrillation.

A prominent J deflection may be present (1).

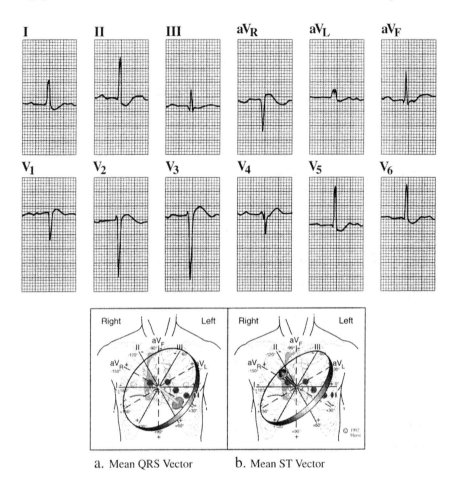

a. Mean QRS Vector   b. Mean ST Vector

Figure 22-1 This electrocardiogram, showing abnormalities due to hypercalcemia plus digitalis effect, was recorded from a 66-year-old woman with severe aortic valve disease, heart failure, and hyperparathyroidism. Her serum calcium level was 12.2 mg/% and her digoxin blood level was 3.2 ng/ml. The P waves are normal and the P-R interval is 0.28 second. The duration of the QRS complexes is 0.08 second. The duration of the Q-T interval is 0.29 second. The S-T segment is short. In *a*, the mean QRS vector is directed at +40° and 70° posteriorly. In *b*, the short S-T segment creates a vector that

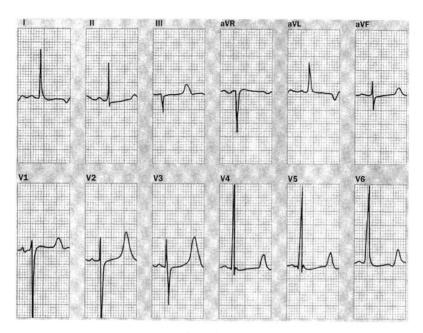

Figure 22-2   This tracing was recorded from a 44-year-old woman with advanced renal failure. The duration of the QT interval is 0.56 second. This prolongation is due to hypocalcemia (a serum calcium of 1.8 mg%). The tent-shaped T waves are the result of hyperkalemia (6.7 mEq/L). The tracing also shows left ventricular hypertrophy. (*Source*: Chung EK. *Cardiac Arrhythmias: Self-Assessment*. Baltimore: Williams & Wilkins, 1977:435. Used with permission.)

---

is quite large. It is directed at about −140° and about 40° anteriorly. The T waves are barely visible. The prolonged P-R interval, short Q-T interval, an S-T segment vector that is directed opposite the mean QRS vector, and small, poorly visible, T wave are typical of digitalis effect. In this example the abnormalities were abetted by hypercalcemia. Ordinarily, it is not wise to administer digitalis to a patient with hypercalcemia (see text). (*Source*: Hurst JW. *Cardiovascular Diagnosis. The Initial Examination*. St. Louis: Mosby-Year Book, Inc, 1993:416. The author, J.W.H., owns the copyright.)

SHORT S-T SEGMENTS IN NORMAL PEOPLE

The Q-T interval may be shorter than usual due to a short S-T segment in otherwise normal subjects. Such individuals may have labile T waves that change considerably with a change in posture, such as standing. As stated in Chapter 23, one wonders if we will discover a short Q-T interval syndrome—there is a definite long Q-T interval syndrome. Might not cardiac arrhythmias be related to *early as well as late* repolarization? It is highly likely that the duration of the S-T segment is determined genetically because it is a component of the Q-T interval, which is determined genetically.

THE ELECTROCARDIOGRAPHIC SIGNS OF HYPOCALCEMIA

The major electrocardiographic sign of hypocalcemia is a long Q-T interval due to prolongation of the S-T segment (see Fig. 22-2).

REFERENCE

1. Gussak I, Bjerregaard P, Egan TM, Chaitman BR. ECG phenomenon called the J wave: history, pathophysiology, and clinical significance. *J Electrocardiol* 1995;28:49–58.

Part VII

Other Abnormalities

Chapter 23

Other Important Electrocardiographic Abnormalities

The electrocardiographic abnormalities discussed in this chapter are usually placed in a book chapter entitled *Miscellaneous*. Placing such electrocardiographic abnormalities in a chapter so titled seems to downgrade the importance of the abnormalities. The abnormalities discussed here are not as common as the signs of ventricular hypertrophy, myocardial infarction, conduction abnormalities, pericarditis, pulmonary disease, digitalis effect, and electrolyte abnormalities, but they must be recognized because most of them are central to the diangosis of *potentially dangerous* cardiac conditions.

PREEXCITATION OF THE VENTRICLES

Electrocardiograms Showing a Short
P-R Interval, Delta Wave, and Prolonged
QRS Duration

Electrocardiograms showing short P-R intervals and prolonged QRS durations were described by Wilson (1), Wedd (2),
and Hamburger (3). In 1930, Wolff, Parkinson, and White reported these abnormalities from patients who experienced episodes of supraventricular tachycardia, but they erroneously
believed the tracings showed a type of bundle branch block (4).
Following this scientific article, many interested physicians
reviewed the tracings in their own files and discovered that
they had previously overlooked the abnormalities. Later, in
1933, Wolfereth and Wood suggested the abnormalities were
due to *preexcitation* of the ventricles rather than bundle
branch block and attributed the condition to an accessory
pathway, such as the bundle of Kent (5). The delta wave itself
was named by Segers, Lequime, and Denolin in 1944 (6).

The electrocardiographic abnormalities of preexcitation
of the ventricles are as follow:

The P-R interval is short. In fact, there is no P-Q interval.
The end of the P wave abuts the beginning of the
QRS complex.

The duration of the QRS complex is 0.09 sec to 0.16 second or longer.

The initial portion of the QRS complex is slurred. This is
called a delta wave because the slant of the wave is
similar to the slant of a Δ wave. This abnormality
may produce abnormal Q waves leading the nascent
interpreter to misdiagnose myocardial infarction.
Two types of delta waves were formerly described:
type A, in which a vector representing the delta wave
was directed anteriorly, and type B, in which a vector representing the delta wave was directed posteriorly (toward the back). Now that we know there are
many types of bypass tracts, the identification of the

exact location of the anomalous pathway is left to the electrophysiologist.

Secondary S-T and T wave abnormalities are usually present.

Patients are prone to experiencing paroxysmal supraventricular tachycardia that is often mistaken for ventricular tachycardia because the QRS complexes are wider than normal. When atrial fibrillation is the rhythm disturbance associated with pre excitation of the ventricles, the ventricular rate may be 220 complexes per minute, which is faster than it is ordinarily. This occurs because the AV node is circumvented in patients who have preexcitation of the ventricles. Despite the rapid ventricular rate, the patient *must not be given digitalis*.

Preexcitation occurs without other evidence of heart disease, but its likelihood is increased in patients with Ebstein's anomaly and in patients with atrial septal defects.

An electrocardiogram showing preexcitation of the ventricles is depicted in Figure 23-1.

SHORT P-R INTERVAL WITH NORMAL QRS DURATION

Lown, Ganong, and Levine (7) reported that patients with short P-R intervals who have normal QRS durations are more likely to have episodes of supraventricular tachycardia than individuals who have P-R intervals that are within the normal range. Recent investigators have denied this relationship, claiming that the short P-R interval is simply part of the normal range of atrioventricular conduction. I am not convinced by their reasoning, because I believe the edges of a bell-shaped curve representing the time required for atrioventricular conduction are overlapped by abnormal atrioventricular conduction times. Therefore, I would argue that a P-R interval of 0.12 second, which is on the part of the bell-shape curve that re-

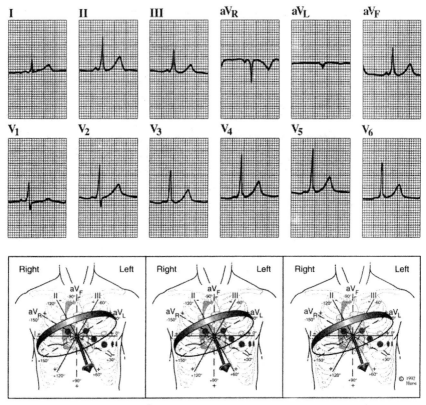

I II III aV_R aV_L aV_F

V₁ V₂ V₃ V₄ V₅ V₆

a. Mean QRS Vector   b. Mean Initial 0.04 Second Vector   c. Mean T Vector

Figure 23-1 This electrocardiogram, showing preexcitation of the QRS complexes, was recorded from a 22-year-old woman who had Wolff-Parkinson-White syndrome. She had experienced episodes of supraventricular tachycardia since she was 6 years of age. Note the short P-R interval and slurred initial forces of the QRS complex (delta wave). The QRS duration is 0.09 second but may be much longer than 0.12 second. The mean QRS vector is directed at about +70° in the frontal plane and 20° or more anteriorly. The vector representing the mean initial 0.04 second QRS complex is directed in a similar direction. Other causes of these QRS abnormalities include true posterior infarction and Duchenne muscular dystrophy. The short P-R interval and delta wave signify the presence of preexcitation of the ventricles. (*Source*: Hurst JW. *Cardiovascular Diagnosis. The Initial Examination*. St. Louis: Mosby-Year Book, Inc, 1993:406. The author, J.W.H., owns the copyright.)

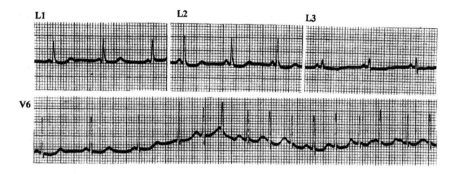

Figure 23-2 This electrocardiogram shows a short P-R interval, but there is no delta wave and the duration of the QRS complexes is 0.07 to 0.08 second. Supraventricular tachycardia is recorded in the lower strip. This condition is referred to as the Lown-Ganong-Levine syndrome (LGL). Many investigators believe that the short P-R normal QRS complex is simply part of the normal range and is not associated with supraventricular tachycardia and that the LGL syndrome does not exist. I am not dissuaded; I believe it does exist. (*Source*: Fisch C. Do you agree? *ACC Current J Review* 1999;8(4): 60. Used with permission.)

flects shorter and shorter P-R intervals, may be normal but can be abnormal in an unspecified percentage of people. Perhaps the James fibers that circumvent the AV node are responsible for this phenomenon in some people. If this is true, the syndrome belongs in a discussion of preexcitation of the ventricles.

An electrocardiogram showing the Lown-Ganong-Levine syndrome is shown in Figure 23-2.

POSTEXCITATION OF THE VENTRICLES

Electrocardiographic Abnormalities Associated with Hypothermia (Osborn Waves)

Although the abnormal deflection due to hypothermia was identified by many earlier observers, it was Osborn's 1953 scientific paper that led the profession to call the deflection an Osborn wave (8). The abnormal wave appears when the body temperature is below 26°C. The abnormal waves are uncommonly caused by conditions other than hypothermia, making it a rather specific abnormality.

The abnormal electrocardiographic abnormalities produced by hypothermia are as follow:

Shiver artifact is commonly present.

Sinus bradycardia, atrial fibrillation, or junctional rhythm may be present.

The duration of the QRS complexes may be 0.16 second or longer.

A spike-and-dome deformity (Osborn wave) may be seen on the downstroke of the QRS complex. This seems to be due to a delayed depolarization of the lateral aspect of the left ventricle. This is the diagnostic feature of the electrocardiogram.

The T waves may become abnormal.

Osborn waves may be seen in persons who are inebriated and sleep outside in the winter, patients in diabetic coma who are exposed to cold weather, and persons who are accidentally exposed to cold weather or simply have no heating system.

An electrocardiogram showing a typical Osborn wave is shown in Figure 23-3.

Postexcitation of the Right Ventricle (Epsilon Waves)

The waves in the electrocardiogram that are characteristic of postexcitation of the right ventricle were identified by Fontaine (9). Fontaine named the waves epsilon because epsilon follows delta in the Greek alphabet and is also a symbol for smallness. The electrocardiographic abnormalities associated with epsilon waves and the characteristics of the waves themselves are listed below.

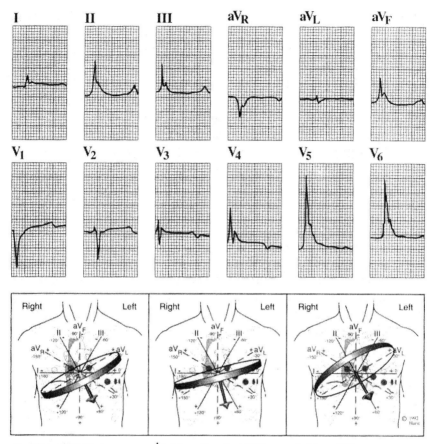

Figure 23-3 This electrocardiogram, showing atrial fibrillation, typical Osborn waves, left ventricular conduction system block, and prolonged Q-T interval, was recorded from a 58-year-old man who had been exposed to low environmental temperature in a poorly run nursing home. He also had pyelonephritis, chronic obstructive lung disease, and a history of prior myocardial infarction. The deformity of the downstroke of the QRS complex is an Osborn wave, which is diagnostic of hypothermia. (*Source*: Top: Clements SD, Hurst JW. Diagnostic value of electrocaridographic abnormalities observed in subjects accidentally exposed to cold. *Am J Cardiol* 1972;29:729. Used with permission. Bottom: Hurst JW. *Cardiovascular Diagnosis. The Initial Examination*. St. Louis: Mosby-Year Book, Inc, 1993: 408. The author, J.W.H., owns the copyright.)

Ventricular tachycardia and ventricular fibrillation may occur.

Epsilon waves are observed in leads V_1 and V_2. They may be seen in leads V_3 and even V_4 when the right ventricle is large. The waves are simply little wiggles in the S-T segments (see Fig. 23-4).

The duration of the QRS complexes in leads V_1 and V_2 may be a little longer than they are in leads V_5 and V_6.

Special Fontaine leads may be used to enhance the little wiggles in the S-T segment (10). These leads are achieved by doubling the sensitivity of the electrocardiograph machine and placing the right arm electrode at the top of the xyphoid, the left arm electrode at the lower end of the sternum, and the left leg electrode at the cardiac apex. The record is then made by recording leads I, II, and III.

Epsilon waves may be recorded from patients with right ventricular dysplasia. The abnormal wiggles in the S-T segment are due to late excitation of myocytes in the right ventricle. Right ventricular dysplasia is characterized by the displacement of myocytes with fat. This delays the excitation and depolarization of the viable myocytes that are enveloped by the fatty tissue, hence the term postexcitation. Epsilon waves can be observed whenever a similar pathological substrate is present. They have been observed in right ventricular infarction, sickle cell anemia with pulmonary hypertension, and rarely in dilated cardiomyopathy.

An electrocardiogram showing epsilon waves is shown in Figure 23-4.

THE BRUGADA SYNDROME

Patients with syncope or proven ventricular tachycardia or fibrillation who usually exhibit right ventricular conduction delay or right bundle branch block and S-T segment elevation

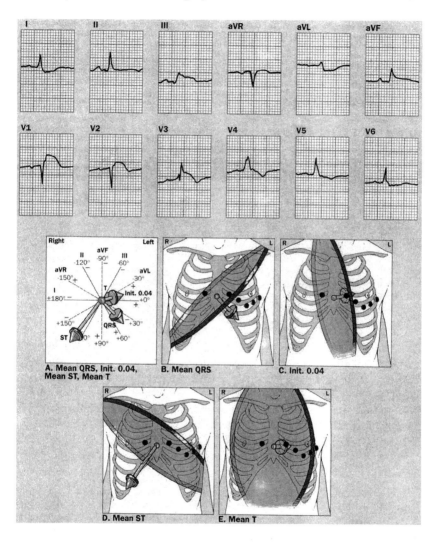

Figure 23-4 This electrocardiogram, showing inferior right ventricular infarction and epsilon waves, was recorded from a 51-year-old man. Note the small wiggles in the S-T segments of V_1 and V_2. Epsilon waves can be recorded in patients with right ventricular dysplasia but can occur whenever viable myocytes on the right ventricle are surrounded by tissue that conducts electrical activity poorly compared to viable myocytes. (*Source:* Hurst JW. *Ventricular Electrocardiography*. New York: Gower Medical Publishing 1991;11.19. The author, J.W.H., owns the copyright.)

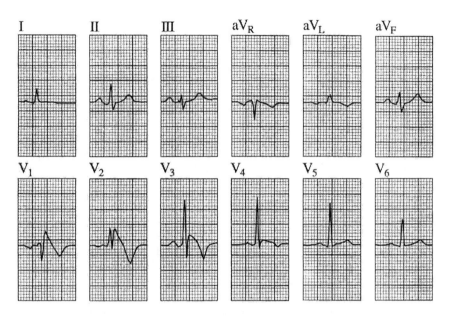

Figure 23-5 This electrocardiogram, showing typical Brugada waves, was recorded from a 31-year-old man who had episodes of ventricular fibrillation. He refused an internal defibrillator and subsequently died. The peculiar S-T segment elevation in leads V_1-V_3 are typical Brugada waves caused by genetically determined abnormal repolarization of the right ventricle (see text). The mean S-T vector is directed anteriorly; there is very little S-T segment displacement in the extremity leads. The mean T vector is directed at +90° in the frontal plane and about 80° posteriorly, representing a repolarization abnormality in the right ventricle. The electrocardiograms of patients with the Brugada syndrome commonly reveal right ventricular conduction delay or right bundle branch block. In this tracing the mean terminal 0.04 QRS vector is directed at −90° in the frontal plane and about 20° to 30° anteriorly, suggesting a delay of the depolarization process in the outflow tract of the right ventricle. (*Source*: This electrocardiogram was provided by Dr. Ihor Gussak, Mayo Physician Alliance for Clinical Trials (MPACT), Mayo Clinic, Rochester, Minnesota.)

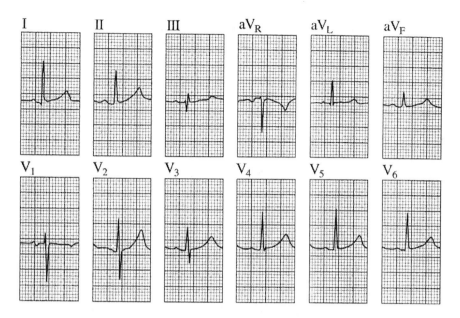

Figure 23-6 This electrocardiogram, showing a long Q-T interval, was recorded from a 10-year-old girl with Jervell-Lange-Nielsen syndrome. Such patients are subject to treacherous ventricular arrhythmias and sudden death. The Q-T interval is 0.40 and the heart rate is 80. The table provided by Ashman and Hull indicates that the normal Q-T interval for a 10-year-old child with a heart rate of 80 is 0.342 second. (*Source*: This tracing was provided by Dr. Arthur Moss of the University of Rochester Medical Center, Rochester, New York.)

in leads V_1-V_3 are said to exhibit the Brugada syndrome (11–14). Gross inspection of the heart reveals no abnormalities. The S-T segment abnormality is due to the loss of the plateau of the dome of the action potential curve. The syndrome is caused by an ion channel gene mutation (5CN5A) (12). The syndrome is being studied actively and it is highly likely that new information will be forthcoming as the months and years pass.

The electrocardiogram recorded from a patient with the Brugada syndrome is shown in Figure 23-5.

LONG QT–SUDDEN DEATH SYNDROME

The long QT–sudden death syndrome has been studied extensively during the past few years. The condition was reported by Jervell-Lange-Nielsen in 1947 (15). Their patients also had congenital deafness. The syndrome was reported in children with normal hearing by Romano in 1963 (16) and Ward in 1964 (17).

The syndrome is characterized by a long Q-T interval, episodes of syncope and ventricular arrhythmias, including ventricular fibrillation that may cause sudden death. Persons with this condition are subject to serious ventricular arrhythmias in response to exercise, anger, or startle. For example, a child with the Romano-Ward syndrome may develop ventricular fibrillation when an alarm clock abruptly awakens him; such individuals with this syndrome are very sensitive to stimulation of the sympathetic nervous system.

Mutations in five genes have been identified in the Romano-Ward syndrome and mutations on two of the genes are responsible for the Jervell and Lange-Nielsen syndrome (18).

The QT interval may be prolonged in newborn babies who subsequently die of what is diagnosed as sudden infant death syndrome (19). This, however, is not the only cause of sudden death in neonates.

An electrocardiogram of a patient with Jervell-Lange-Neilsen syndrome is shown in Figure 23-6.

REFERENCES

1. Wilson FN. A case in which the vagus influenced the form of the ventricular complex of the electrocardiogram. Arch Intern Med 1915;16:1008–1027.

2. Wedd AM. Paroxysmal tachycardia; with reference to nomo-

topic tachycardia and the role of the extrinsic cardiac nerves. Arch Intern Med 1921;27:571–590.

3. Hamburger WW. Bundle-branch block: 4 cases of intraventricular block showing some interesting and unusual clinical features. Med Clin North Am 1929;13:343–362.

4. Wolff L, Parkinson J, White PD. Bundle-branch block with the short P-R interval in healthy young people prone to paroxysmal tachycardia. Am Heart J 1930;5:685–704.

5. Wolferth CC, Wood FC. The mechanism of production of short P-R intervals and prolonged QRS complexes in patients with presumably undamaged hearts: hypothesis of an accessory pathway of auriculoventricular conduction (bundle of Kent). Am Heart J 1933;8:297–311.

6. Segers PM, Lequime J, Denolin H. L'activation ventriculaire précoce de certains coeurs hyperexcitables: etude de l'onde Δ de l'électrocardiogramme. Cardiologia 1944;8:113–167.

7. Lown B, Ganong WF, Levine SA. The syndrome of short P-R interval, normal QRS complex, and paroxysmal rapid heart action. Circulation 1952;5:693.

8. Osborn JJ. Experimental hypothermia: respiratory and blood pH changes in relation to cardiac function. Am J Physiol 1953; 175:389–398.

9. Hurst JW. Naming of the waves in the ECG, with a brief account of their genesis. Circulation 1998;98:1941.

10. Hurst JW. Naming of the waves in the ECG, with a brief account of their genesis. Circulation 1998;98:1940.

11. Brugada P, Brugada J. Right bundle branch block, persistent ST segment elevation and sudden cardiac death: A distinct clinical and electrocardiographic syndrome. A multicenter report. J Am Coll Cardiol 1992;20:1391–1396.

12. Gussak I, Bjerregard P, Antzelevitch C, Towbin J, Chaitman BR. The Brugada syndrome: clinical, electrophysiologic, and genetic aspects. J Am Coll Cardiol 1999;33:5–15.

13. Miyazaki T, Mitamura H, Miyoshi S, et al. Autonomic and anti-

arrhythmic drug modulation of ST segment elevation in patients with Brugada syndrome. J Am Coll Cardiol 1996;27:
1061–70.

14. Chen Q, Kirsch GE, Zhang D, Brugada R, Brugada, J, Brugada
    P, et al. Genetic basis and molecular mechanisms for idiopathic
    ventricular fibrillation. Nature 1998;392:293–296.

15. Jervell A, Lange-Nielsen F. Congenital deaf mutism, functional
    heart disease with prolongation of the QT interval, and sudden
    death. Am Heart J 1947;54:59–68.

16. Romano C, Gemme G, Pongiglione R. Arithmie cardiache rare
    dell'eta pediatrica. Clin Pediatr 1963;45:656–683.

17. Ward OC. A new familial cardiac syndrome in children. J Irish
    Med Assoc 1964;54:103–106.

18. Splawski I, Jiaxiang S, Timothy KW, et al. Spectrum of muta-
    tions in long-QT syndrome genes. Circulation 2000;102:1178–
    1185.

19. Schwartz PJ, Stramba-Badiale M, Seganti A, et al. Prolonga-
    tion of the QT interval and the sudden infant death syndrome.
    N Engl J Med 1998;338:1709–1714.

Part VIII

Conclusion

Chapter 24

Final Comment

Interpreting electrocardiograms is like multiplying. It is possible to memorize single-digit multiplication, but when we attempt to multiply double- or triple-digit numbers we find that our memory fails us. We accomplish the act of multiplying double- or triple-digit numbers by *using a system* that reduces the double or triple digits to single digits. So, as with multiplying, the brain cannot memorize all the different electrocardiographic abnormalities, this book emphasizes *a system of basic principles, including the use of vectors, that should be used to interpret each electrocardiogram.*

Some people learn to diagram vectors with precision and then memorize vector patterns. If the reader falls into that trap, then I have failed in my efforts. Should this be the case, the reader is advised to review the images, or memories, presented in Chapters 3 through 8. These images, or memories, must be reviewed again and again until they are permanently stored in the working memory. When possible, as repeatedly emphasized, these memories should be linked to other memories that are already stored in the memory bank of the brain. The point is, if memorization is used, it should be directed toward the memorization and storage of basic principles, rather than trying to memorize all the different electrocardiographic patterns. It is not uncommon for an early learner to ask, "Will you show us a few electrocardiograms?" I usually respond, "You can't learn electrocardiography that way. I will be delighted to discuss some of the basic principles that are required to interpret electrocardiograms. In due time, when you have mastered the principles, I will show you hundreds of tracings."

Finally, after learning the basic principles needed to interpret each electrocardiogram, the individual responsible for analyzing the tracings must become fluent. Fluency is developed by decreasing the time required for the thought process used to interpret tracings. Therefore, the interpreter must increase the speed used to call up the memories discussed in Chapters 3 through 8, determine the anatomic-electrophysiological differential diagnosis, create a differential diagnosis indicating the cardiac diseases the patient might have, and correlate the electrocardiographic interpretation with the other clinical data.

Finally, I do not wish to convey the idea that the use of the approach described in this book will solve all problems. I do believe it will solve more problems than can be solved by memorizing the shapes of deflection. The method of interpretation described here will also identify some electrocardiographic problems that cannot be explained. Even that is better than not recognizing that the problems exists, which is likely when the memory system is used.

I have found the approach discussed here to be exciting because it brings a degree of satisfaction and enjoyment to the interpretative effort. When the electrocardiographic abnormalities fit the other abnormalities, the diagnostic puzzle is solved. This correlative act should be as exciting as reading the final chapter of a well-written detective story in which the guilty one is identified and all the clues fit. On the other hand, when the electrocardiographic diagnosis does not fit the other data collected from the patient, the intellectual pursuit must continue because the patient either has two different types of heart disease or the data collection process has been imperfect. This, too, is like a detective story in which the clues do not fit. In such a case, the detective reexamines the data he or she has already collected and searches for new and different clues.

Index

About the Author

J. WILLIS HURST is a Consultant to the Division of Cardiology, Emory University School of Medicine, Atlanta, Georgia, where he was professor and chairman of the Department of Medicine from 1957 to 1986. The author or coauthor of more than 60 books, including *Clinical Neurocardiology* (Marcel Dekker, Inc.), and nearly 400 articles devoted to scientific medicine, Dr. Hurst is a member of the American Heart Association and the American College of Cardiology, and was selected Master of the American College of Physicians. He received the B.S. degree (1941) from the University of Georgia, Atlanta, and the M.D. degree (1944) from the Medical College of Georgia, Augusta, and was a cardiology fellow with Dr. Paul White at Massachusetts General Hospital, Boston.

Chiu

= Ashman's phenom

< LVH ?? Septal infarct
Pseud.